OXFORD MED

Palliative Care Ethics

Palliative Care Ethics

A Companion for all Specialties

Second Edition

FIONA RANDALL

Consultant in Palliative Medicine
Bournemouth and Christchurch Hospital Trust

and

R. S. DOWNIE

Professor of Moral Philosophy
Glasgow University

OXFORD
UNIVERSITY PRESS

OXFORD
UNIVERSITY PRESS

Oxford University Press, Great Clarendon Street, Oxford OX2 6DP

Oxford New York
Athens Auckland Bangkok Bogotá Buenos Aires Calcutta
Cape Town Chennai Dar es Salaam Delhi Florence Hong Kong Istanbul
Karachi Kuala Lumpur Madrid Melbourne Mexico City Mumbai
Nairobi Paris São Paulo Singapore Taipei Tokyo Toronto Warsaw
and associated companies in
Berlin Ibadan

Oxford is a trade mark of Oxford University Press

Published in the United States
by Oxford University Press, Inc., New York

First Edition published 1996
Reprinted 1996, 1998
Second Edition published 1999

A catalogue record for this book is available from the British Library

Library of Congress Cataloging in Publication Data
Randall, Fiona
Palliative care ethics : a companion for all specialties / Fiona
Randall and R.S. Downie. – 2nd ed.
Includes bibliographical references and index.
1. Palliative treatment–Moral and ethical aspects. 2. Palliative
treatment–Decision making. 3. Terminal care–Moral and ethical
aspects. 4. Terminal care–Decision making. I. Downie, R. S.
(Robert Silcock) II. Title.
[DNLM: 1. Confidentiality. 2. Decision Making. 3. Ethics,
Medical. 4. Palliative Care. 5. Physician-Patient Relations.
W50 R188p 1999]
R726.R35 1999   362.1'75–dc21   99-20410

ISBN 0 19 263068 7 (Pbk : alk. paper)

Typeset by Downdell, Oxford
Printed in Great Britain
on acid-free paper by
Biddles Ltd.
Guildford and King's Lynn

If the changes we fear be thus irresistible, what remains but to acquiesce with silence, as in the other insurmountable distresses of humanity? It remains that we retard what we cannot repel, that we palliate what we cannot cure.

Samuel Johnson (1755)
from *A Dictionary of the English Language*

Foreword

Dr Derek Doyle,
St Columba's Hospice, Edinburgh

Some topics feature so frequently in specialist palliative care that one might perhaps be forgiven for believing they are almost unique to this work. Closer observation, however, reveals that they are merely brought into sharper focus in the field of palliative care but are central issues to the whole practice of medicine. They include such topics as communication, 'whole person care' as it has come to be termed, quality of life, research issues, and the subject of this book—ethical issues. Clearly to regard them as unique to, or only important in, palliative care would be both wrong and insulting to many colleagues in other specialties and disciplines for they are of equal relevance to us all. Perhaps it is the nature of our work as palliative care specialists which makes them such common topics of conversation and concern. However, this does not necessarily make us more knowledgeable or expert in them. Rather are we made more painfully aware of our lack of training and understanding in these and so many other areas and find ourselves searching for expert guidance.

I feel honoured to be counted amongst those who encouraged the authors of this book to write it for our guidance. We recognized their unquestionable qualification to do so, and the urgency with which they have had to work, as palliative care is so rapidly developing not only in the United Kingdom but worldwide, and identical ethical considerations are challenging its practitioners almost everywhere. As the authors are themselves so clearly aware, palliative care is the right of all who suffer and die from whatever pathology, only a few of them needing specialist care. Just as the principles of relieving physical suffering apply to them all wherever they are, whatever their mortal illness, so the imperative to study and understand the underlying ethical issues applies to every doctor and nurse committed to serving them, whatever their specialty, in whatever country they practise. Though such things as the Patient's Charter and the Community Care Act may appear uniquely British, in fact similar principles or laws are in force in many countries where also may be found market-place economies, grave financial constraints, limited resources, and competing priorities, all topics addressed in this book.

It would be dishonest to claim that most of us find the study and discussion of ethics easy. We do not. It is tempting and foolish to protest, as many have done, that ethics is either 'common sense' or so abstract a subject that it is best left to the philosophers whilst we the clinicians get on with our work, well intentioned but without much ethical framework. If this book does not more than illustrate the centrality of ethics to all we do, it will have justified all the work that has gone into it but, I have not the slightest doubt, it will achieve much more than that. No longer will anyone be able to think that the key ethical issues in medicine are euthanasia, advance directives, patient-assisted death, and persistent vegetative state, as the media would have us believe. As if to highlight this the authors have, rightly in my view, chosen not to address some of these, feeling they have been adequately dealt with in other texts. Rather they focused on matters of *daily* relevance such as clinical decision making, patient autonomy, nurse advocacy, the needs of relatives and fellow professionals in the care team, information giving and sharing, confidentiality, and quality of care.

It is often said that a metaphorical halo shines over specialist palliative care and its practitioners with the result that some of its claims and assumptions have gone unchallenged by all but a few. It is, for example, rarely questioned whether we have as much right to involve ourselves in spiritual issues as we have in physical and psychological suffering. We speak of truth telling, and often pride ourselves on having the courage and the skill to do so when others may have shirked it, without pausing to ask how much the patient wants to know. We speak of relatives and their needs as being as much the focus of our care as the dying patient but rarely ask if this is ethically right. Each day we make important clinical decisions without giving sufficient thought to the decision-making process , so confident are we that we always know what is right for our patients. We pride ourselves on our teamwork, seeing it as a model which could and should be adopted by other health care professionals but perhaps we also need to be challenged about this central feature of specialist palliative care.

How helpful to be reminded by the authors that the term 'total good' is a more useful one than 'holistic' and that our commitment to it is *intrinsic* to our role as carers; that we have intrinsic aims such as the relief of physical and psychological suffering but that attention to social and spiritual needs is an *extrinsic* aim. Some will predictably be disturbed by their assertion that we do not have an indisputable right to question and probe into every shadowy corner of a family, nor to describe to a patient every therapeutic option when some are irrelevant—though they should be told at least as much about their illness as they wish to know. Whoever we are, palliative care specialists, oncologists, surgeons, physicians, or nurses, we need to be reminded that treatment options should be selected on the basis of benefits to burdens/risks calculus, a principle so obvious that we are left wondering why we were not trained to use this in practice. Many clinicians will find themselves indebted to these authors but one cannot help hoping that the book will be read by those who have designed the Patient's Charter and the Community Care Act, both of which the authors find good reason to challenge, and also by managers who would be reminded that some essential aspects of palliative care are not measurable in numerical terms but must be assessed in qualitative terms which entail value judgements. How helpful to see it stated, 'It is not morally acceptable to omit them because they cannot be evaluated numerically'.

Dare we hope that one of their key conclusions will be taken to heart by us all, whoever we are ... 'Palliative care needs well developed, wise, and compassionate people, whose common sense is combined with professional knowledge; it does not need people who lack these characteristics but are trained to appear as if they possess them.'

We who now have this book are truly in the debt of its authors who so clearly are well developed, wise, compassionate, and full of common sense. Palliative care will be the richer for their wisdom.

Preface to the second edition

In the first edition of *Palliative Care Ethics* our subtitle was *A Good Companion*. In what follows we explain what we meant by this subtitle. In this second edition our approach is the same. Nevertheless, we have made a slight change to the subtitle. The reason for the change is to stress that palliative care is not a separate self-contained specialty but is an integral part of most specialties. It is a fact of human existence that we all die and in the time leading up to our death we are likely to be treated and cared for by general practitioners, general physicians, oncologists, nurses, and so on. Ethical problems of the sort we discuss are likely to occur in any of these spheres of health care, and we hope our book will be relevant and helpful to all health care practitioners.

There are other significant changes in the second edition. New examples have been added throughout and also a discussion of the special issues of consent in palliative care, but more importantly there are three new chapters. First, we have added a chapter on 'The relative–professional relationship'. Traditionally, the central relationship in health care is between the patient and the professional. But increasingly, and especially in palliative care, relatives wish to be involved, not just to receive appropriate information but to influence treatment decisions.

Those in charge of palliative care must of course be good companions to relatives. This is true of every area of health care. One special problem for palliative care, however, arises if the patient's relatives are given an almost equal priority with patients in the remit. How realistic or desirable is this? Is it realistic to expect staff with limited resources to be equally concerned with both the patient and the relatives? Time is a limited resource and it should not be given to relatives at the expense of patients. Moreover, it is not desirable to turn the grief and bereavement of relatives into professional problems. Most people can cope with their own emotions, however painful. But there is a widespread tendency in society to professionalize every problem and so de-skill ordinary people. Such attitudes are patronizing and destructive of good companionship.

There is another danger in including relatives in the remit of palliative care, namely that relatives may acquire too big a say in the treatment of the patient. If the patient is autonomous, then treatment decisions should be reached after consultation with the patient rather than the relatives, although obviously relatives need a say if they are going to be involved in the care. If the patient is not autonomous, then the opinion of the relatives is important, but what must remain paramount in that situation is the professional's own judgement. Companionship with relatives should not compromise professionalism.

Secondly, we have added a chapter in which we reply to our critics. Points of importance were raised by critics. In particular, we are glad to have the opportunity to expand on an ethical issue which we first raised in Chapter 1, but which has developed in a marked manner since the appearance of the first edition—the rise of 'respect for patient autonomy' as the supreme and over-riding ethical principle. We cannot wholly endorse this one-gun approach to ethics. Again, in this new chapter we offer an extended discussion of topical issues raised by some critics—withholding and withdrawing treatment, and intending and foreseeing outcomes. Some critics wish to attach these issues to euthanasia. A logical attachment of this sort can give rise to two sorts of argument. If withholding and withdrawing treatment leads to or is a form of euthanasia, and the former are ethically appropriate, then so should the latter be ethically appropriate. Alternatively, it can be argued that since euthanasia is not ethically appropriate, then withholding and withdrawing treatment cannot be either. We avoid this argument by denying the premise—that there is a logical connection between withholding and withdrawing, or intending and foreseeing, and active voluntary euthanasia.

Finally, we have added a chapter on 'The quality and value of life'. In all our other chapters we have attempted to stay close to the clinical situation. But it can be a failing of all those working in health care that they remain too close to the clinical situation, and as a result cannot see the wood for the trees. What we have tried to do in this last chapter is to offer a much broader philosophical view of the concepts of quality and value of life. We hope that this chapter will provide a fresh perspective on the ethical issues of the clinical situation.

We have said that we hope our book will be a good ethical companion to those involved in the palliative end of any specialty. Let us now expand on what we mean by calling our book a 'companion'.

On one level we intend simply to convey that the book is offered as an ethical companion to *The Oxford Textbook of Palliative Medicine. The Oxford Textbook* does indeed contain a chapter on ethics, but that is mainly concerned with euthanasia. Euthanasia is not part of palliative care however, although the subject may sometimes arise in that context. On the other hand, there are many other issues, less commonly discussed, which are part of palliative care; it is these we address. We hope that our book will be a good companion to the doctors, nurses, and other members of the health care team facing these issues.

On another level the title is intended to remind professionals that they should be good companions to patients. Now in one sense this reminder is totally unnecessary, for palliative care by its very nature is concerned with support and companionship in the last stages of life, rather than with heroic rescue attempts and cures. But there are ethical dangers here. Emotional and spiritual care and companionship may seem such incontestably good things that they are never scrutinized in the manner of physical care. Yet some patients may not want the attention of counsellors or spiritual advisers, or wish in any way to discuss intimate matters with professional staff. Being a good companion to patients then means ensuring that there has been consent to emotional care.

But there is another strand to our argument on this matter. In what may be a controversial aspect of the book, we argue that there cannot be a specifically professional expertise in emotional care. Of course, there is such a thing as clinical depression and no doubt there is a professional expertise to help with this. But the normal fears, anxieties, regrets, or guilt of human beings facing their death are not appropriate subjects for professional techniques. Indeed, there is no genuine expertise in this area. Does this mean that palliative care has nothing to offer patients in their distress? Certainly not! Our thesis is that there can be no *professional* expertise, not that nothing can be offered. What can and ought to be offered if the patient seeks it, is the comfort and reassurance that can come from the company of a warm and balanced personality.

In pursuing this theme we shall argue that professional expertise can never be a substitute for the humane insights of the carer. Palliative care requires mature and balanced professionals with a broad experience of life. In other areas of health care we hear of problems becoming 'over-medicalized'. There is less danger of that in palliative care. But there is a danger of problems becoming 'over-psychologized'. Balanced judgements are necessary and they are more likely to be made by someone with broad interests. As J. S. Mill (1859) put it:

> It really is of importance not only what men do, but also what manner of men they are that do it.

But how can staff develop in themselves warm personalities and balanced judgement? How can they become not just expert professionals but good companions? The answer (well, the start of the answer) is that they should not be too hard on themselves! There is a tendency for those in health care to drive themselves unsparingly into long hours of work. But this practice can have bad outcomes for staff and patients. As C. S. Lewis (1942) put it:

> She's the sort of woman who lives for others—you can always tell the others by their hunted expressions.

In other words, we think it important that those who work in the demanding and stressful specialty of palliative care should cultivate interests well outside their work. This is partly for their own sakes— to avoid becoming stale or even burned out—but also so that they may be good companions to their patients.

The book is divided very roughly into three parts. Chapters 1–5 are the more general and express our basic philosophy of palliative care, Chapters 6–12 deal with a range of clinical topics, and Chapters 13 and 14 raise wider and more challenging philosophical issues. While we have endeavoured to integrate every topic into a coherent whole, the chapters should be intelligible separately to those who have specific interests within the general area of palliative care. We have tried to fuse theory and practice with the aim of providing an overall philosophy of palliative care which will be at the same time practically relevant and intellectually challenging. The detailed discussions of issues in palliative care have been linked to wider human concerns by prefacing each chapter with a brief literary quotation. We hope that these quotations will bring out that there is more to ethical issues than can be demonstrated by argument. The majority of these quotations are taken from *The Healing Arts: An Oxford Illustrated Anthology*, edited by R. S. Downie (1994), Oxford University Press.

Christchurch   F. R.
Glasgow   R. S. D.
February 1999

Acknowledgements

We are grateful to Oxford University Press for pointing out the need for a book on palliative care ethics written primarily from a clinical point of view. The Royal Bournemouth and Christchurch Hospital Trust generously provided sabbatical leave which enabled amorphous discussions to be turned into draft chapters. We are grateful to Mr Jonathan Montgomery of the Faculty of Law of Southampton University, who has advised us on legal matters, and to Anne Southall, Anne Valentine, and Susan Stone for secretarial help. Dr Derek Doyle of St Columba's Hospice, Edinburgh, has drawn on a lifetime of practical experience to advise us on many issues and to write a foreword. Finally, our respective spouses have had to put up with the rows between us which were generated by this collaboration. We thank them for their forbearance and hope our readers will be stimulated not into rows but into reflecting on this important area of health care.

Contents

1

Ethics and aims in palliative care

Nothing is fixed in matters of conduct and of what is useful, any more than in matters of health. Since even the general account is like this, the account of particular cases is still less exact. The cases do not fall under any art or precept. Instead the agents themselves must all the time consider what is appropriate to the particular occasion, just as in medicine or navigation.

Aristotle, from *Nicomachean Ethics*

In the opening chapter we shall begin by introducing the ethical concepts and principles which are used in contemporary discussions of health care. We shall then go on to discuss the aims of palliative care, relating them to the general aims of health care. Finally, we shall put the ethics and the aims together and show how these are integrated. It will emerge that to adopt the aims of palliative care is to adopt a moral standpoint.

1.1 The senses of 'ethics'

In recent years health care professionals, and the public they serve, have become more conscious of the complexity of the moral problems which can be created by caring for other people. There is now growing awareness of the need to identify clearly what these moral problems are, and to arrive at possible solutions for the patients and for the nurses, doctors, or other professionals concerned, while taking into account wider social issues.

An initial complication is that problems in health care have traditionally been identified as 'ethical' rather than 'moral' and there has developed the mistaken idea that there are special kinds of expertise called 'medical ethics' and 'nursing ethics', and correspondingly that those who care for others have special claims to knowing or deciding what is right and wrong in health and illness.

Moreover, by being members of a profession concerned with the well-being of people, doctors in particular, but also nurses and other health care workers, have allowed themselves to be seen as arbiters in public and private moral dilemmas for which they may have no more expertise than any other thoughtful and considerate person. On the other hand, those who care for others do have special kinds of non-moral knowledge and the experience of dealing with those who are seriously ill—that knowledge and experience does give them some claim to be listened to and will certainly affect their moral or ethical decisions. What is helpful is that those who care for us when we are ill should have some familiarity with the arguments and concepts which are employed in ethical discussion.

There is a second source of confusion which must be removed at the start—the term 'ethics' is ambiguous. First, 'ethics' can refer to that branch of philosophy also called 'moral philosophy'. Ethics in this sense is a theoretical study of practical morality and its aim is to discover, analyse, and relate to each other the fundamental concepts and principles of ordinary practical morality.

The second main sense of 'ethics' is ordinary morality or value judgements as they are found in a professional context. This usage brings out the *continuity* between the moral problems of everyday life and those encountered in hospitals or other spheres of professional practice. Morality or ethics must be seen broadly as including the whole area of value judgements about good and harm.

The third sense of 'ethics' refers to codes of procedure, or ethics narrowly conceived. These are important for they give some of the principles which underlie professional activity and they apply across cultural and national boundaries.

It is worthwhile stressing the difference between the second broad sense of ethics as value judgement and the narrow sense which refers simply to the items on a traditional list. For example, in the wide sense it is a moral or value judgement that a given patient, all factors considered, ought to be allowed home despite the risk of a recurrence of his or her problem. But clearly this decision does not raise a question of morality or ethics narrowly conceived. It is because many health care professions take ethics or morality in the narrow sense that they are unaware of the extent to which they are continually making moral or value judgements in the broad sense. There are certainly technical—scientific and social—factors involved in deciding whether or not a given patient ought to be allowed home. But the decision about what in the end ought to be done goes beyond the technical and encompasses the professional's overall judgement as to what is for the total good of the patient. This overall, all things considered, judgement of the patient's good is what we mean by a moral or value judgement. One of the central aims of teaching ethics is to make the professional aware of the all-pervasive nature of such value judgements and the extent to which the professional's own values affect decisions.

1.2 The main tradition

From the time of Hippocrates until the 1960s medical ethics was seen in terms of doctors' duties to patients. These duties have traditionally been thought of as those of not harming the patient (non-maleficence) and of helping the patient (beneficence). Under-lying these two apparently simple types of duty there are, however, complexities. Medical understanding of these duties has been affected by three different currents of thinking. Let us examine these currents, which are discussed by Jonsen (1990).

The first current is the one flowing from the origins of modern medicine in the Greek world. When the Hippocratic Oath requires the physician not to harm but to help, it is against a background of Greek craftsmanship. The art or craft (*techne*) of the carpenter is to work on wood according to the nature of wood. There are bounds or limits concerning what is appropriate for each craft, and to go beyond these bounds is to be guilty of *hubris* or pride. Hence, when the Greek doctor promises not to harm and to do good to the patient, what is intended is much the same requirement as that laid on the carpenter when, as a good craftsman, he tries not to damage his material, wood, but rather to bring out its nature as wood. We might term the Hippocratic ethic that of the competent craftsman. The relevant portion of the Hippocratic Oath really indicates that there are constraints on the skill or art of medicine; it does not truly involve beneficence in our modern sense.

But beneficence in our modern sense enters the scene via the Samaritan tradition in medicine. It is known that St Luke was a physician and there is some evidence that the good Samaritan was meant to be a physician—certainly he treats the man fallen by the wayside with an infundation of oil and wine, which was a remedy for wounds in Greek medicine. However that may be, the ideal of the good Samaritan who ministers to the sick despite inconvenience and danger to himself was one which enormously affected the tradition of medicine, and it gave us the ideal of beneficence in something like its modern form.

Yet not completely like its form in modern medicine, for another current also affected medical beneficence. Historians of medicine have debated about the origins of this tradition, but it may have been in the religious orders which were founded to care for the sick and wounded during the Crusades. For example, the Order of Knights Hospitallers was founded in the eleventh century to provide hostels for pilgrims to the Holy Land and to care for the sick, and later those wounded at the Crusades. The members of this Order were mainly of noble families and were dedicated to serve 'our lords, the sick' (a favourite phrase). This tradition continued in the religious orders, and it emerged in a different form in the eighteenth century when the status and education of doctors began once again to improve, and the image of the gentleman-physician began to reappear. The opening words of the influential book of medical ethics, written by the British physician Thomas Percival (1803), bear witness in elegant language to the ethic of *noblesse oblige*:

Physicians and surgeons should minister to the sick, reflecting that the ease, health and lives of those committed to their charge depend on their skills, attention and fidelity. They should study, in their deportment, so to unite tenderness with steadiness, and condescension with authority, as to inspire the minds of their patients with gratitude, respect and confidence.

These words echo the sentiments of the Knights Hospitallers of the Crusades, and they were incorporated into the Code of Ethics of the American Medical Association and stood unchanged from 1847 to 1912; their spirit lived long after that.

To sum this up, we can say that all doctors would nowadays subscribe to the ethical idea that they have duties not to harm and to do good to their patients, but they may be unaware of the fact that the medical interpretation of these duties has been coloured by (at least) three traditions: the Hippocratic tradition of competent craftsmanship, the Samaritan tradition of helping one's neighbour in all circumstances, and the Knights Hospitallers' tradition of noble service.

This rich medical ethos, which we shall call 'the main tradition', remained largely undisturbed from the Greek world to the end of the 1950s. Since then, however, there have been at least three attacks on it, deriving from three different sets of ideas: the emergence of nursing as an independent profession and along with that the development of a team approach to health care; the rise of patients' rights movements; and the need for rationing following the growth of demand on medical services. These movements overlap in various ways, and all are particular manifestations of broader social changes.

1.3 Teams and the nursing profession

The demand for a team approach to health care has been greatly influenced by the rise of nursing to full professional status. Nurses are nowadays very intolerant of the traditional references of doctors to 'my' patients. They are increasingly demanding consultation before important decisions affecting patient care are taken. Hence we have one partial explanation of the increasing use of teams making joint decisions. Other parts of the explanation—such as the increasingly technical complexity of the decisions which therefore require a range of specialist opinion—do not concern us here. But granted that nursing opinion is increasingly important in decisions, we find the beginnings of a new approach to health care which involves more group decisions. The emergence of group decision making (and the extent of it varies a great deal) is therefore a challenge to the older ideas of the doctors' duties. Let us hope that if there can be broad discussion involving not only different specialists but also different gender perspectives, more balanced decision may result. Before leaving this topic, however, we should note that group decision making involves group responsibility. If nursing wishes as a profession to have equal claim to be heard with doctors, then nurses must be willing to be held responsible for their decisions (see Chapter 4).

Although the rise of other professional groups and the consequent challenge to (predominantly) male medical supremacy in decision making has perhaps been psychologically disturbing to the medical profession, there is no reason why it cannot be assimilated into the traditional approach to patient care. Instead of thinking of the

supremacy of medical duties to patients we can think of team-based
duties and hope that the decisions of a broadly based team are more
compassionate and less 'gung-ho' then they otherwise might have
been. But this is a development and humanizing of the great tradition
rather than an abandonment of it. We shall follow contemporary
practice and refer, as from Chapter 2, to 'health care ethics' rather
than 'medical ethics'.

1.4   Patients' rights and autonomy

A more radical challenge to the tradition may be thought to come
from the appearance of the patients' rights movement. This movement is not unconnected with the rise of nursing as a profession,
because many nurses see themselves as what they call 'the patient's
advocate', where what they are advocating is that patients' rights
should be observed. But the patients' rights movement is influenced
by many other considerations. One broad influence has been the
general democratization of society in the post-war period. The
public in general terms wish to be involved in decisions which are
going to affect them. This move to more openness, more consultation, has affected medicine as much as other branches of society.
More specifically, within medicine the rise of patients' rights
movements was influenced by the exposure of abuses in medical
research, when it emerged in the 1960s that in some cases informed
consent was not being obtained for dangerous research. The result
was that, first in the United States and then in the United Kingdom,
research ethics committees were established, and this in turn
influenced the medical approach to the doctor–patient relationship. The concept which has been adopted to encapsulate the idea of
the rights of patients is 'autonomy'. Codes of medical ethics and
philosophical discussion from the 1970s increasingly added 'respect
for the patient's autonomous decisions' to the duties of non-
maleficence and beneficence. Around the same period the concept of
justice was brought into play. This sometimes seemed to mean
treating individual patients justly, say by observing their rights, and
sometimes that autonomous patients were all equally entitled to
equal shares in the distribution of health care. For almost two
decades discussions of medical ethics have been conducted in the US
and the UK very largely in terms of the four principles of non-

maleficence, beneficence, respect for autonomy, and justice, and many influential text-books have been written, and indeed are still being written, using them as the necessary and sufficient principles of humane discussion in medical ethics.

Before going on to examine the principle of respect for autonomy in more detail, we should perhaps fill out slightly more of the philosophical position. The four principles can be seen, and were seen by the majority of writers, as first-order moral principles, to be used in reaching medical decisions when ethical questions were raised. It is a separate matter, and one for the moral philosopher, how these principles can be justified. Are they each an expression of a single underlying principle or are they each independently valid, and if so what happens if they clash? These and many related matters are the concern of moral philosophy proper, and we do not intend to pursue them in this book. But it is worth noting, for the terms are often used in ethical debate, that those who think that there is a single underlying principle often identify that principle as the principle of utility—that actions are right if they maximize individual preferences, or in older terminology, if they bring about the greatest happiness of the greatest number. As opposed to the utilitarians, those who hold that the principles can each independently be seen to be valid have been called 'deontologists'. We shall not pursue the interesting debates which have clustered round these theories.

Returning to the principle of respect for the patient's autonomy we shall find that once we look beyond the slogan it is not clear what is meant by 'autonomy'. There are in fact at least two ways of interpreting it. One interpretation is compatible with what we are calling 'the main tradition' of medical ethics and is an enrichment of it, but the second is not compatible, and indeed it implies a radical change in the doctor–patient relationship.

The idea of 'autonomy', of persons as self-determining, self-governing beings, is first discussed with a proper understanding of what it means by Kant (1785). He assumes that people are essentially rational, although our desires may at times blind us. Decisions which are made as a result of dominant or blinding desires he called 'heteronomous'. They are not truly the desires of the self, for they are caused by the non-rational aspects of human nature.

The Kantian tradition of moral philosophy as it affected medical ethics was modified by the liberal tradition of J. S. Mill (1859). Briefly, Mill argues that we have a right to do whatever we want unless it can be shown that we are harming others. The key difference between Kant's approach to autonomy and Mill's lies in the respective emphases given to rationality and preferences. For Kant, a decision is autonomous if it is rational (whether it expresses our preferences or not). For Mill, an autonomous decision does express our preference and it is less important whether the decision is rational. These traditions have merged and what has come out is autonomy as the expression of informed preferences or consent to whatever we do or is done to us by others.

This fused Kantian–Millean conception of autonomy, as preference or as informed consent, is one which can be absorbed by what we are terming the main tradition. No doubt the doctor–patient relationship always involved some sort of consultation and discussion, and we can read the more recent emphasis on autonomy, on obtaining informed consent for all medical decisions, as an extension of and an insistence on that process of consultation. It can be seen as an antidote to the paternalism which was the pathology of the doctor–patient relationship in the past, and as a way of modernizing the relationship, of modifying it in terms of the modern ethos of openness in human relationship. It is important to note, however, that autonomous choice or informed consent in this sense takes place within the context of a professional consultation, with the patient retaining the right of veto to unwanted treatment and the doctor retaining the right of veto to treatment professionally considered useless or harmful. But now let us look at the important difference when preference autonomy becomes consumer autonomy.

To set the scene consider a genuine situation of consumer autonomy. Suppose that a person goes into a shoe shop and asks for a pair of strong shoes for walking along country lanes. He tries on various pairs which do not appeal to him and then his eye lights on a pair of shiny patent leather shoes and he says he wants to buy them. A good salesperson will explain to him that they are not appropriate shoes for his purposes, but if he insists that these are the ones he wants the salesperson has no duty to refuse the sale having advised against it. The customer here is exercising consumer autonomy. Can this idea be carried over into the medical context? Many ethicists think that it can, and indeed the British Government is encouraging the idea of consumer autonomy in health care to the extent that patients are being exhorted to see themselves as customers. Let us look at the ethics literature on this.

Take the situation in which a patient, or relatives of the patient, request treatment which the doctor believes is useless or even harmful. In a study surveying the literature on this, Paris *et al.* (1993) note that doctors will almost always continue treatment if requested by patients or relatives even if they regard it as futile. They do this because they believe that patient autonomy carries with it the right to whatever treatment the patient requests. Moreover, this view is supported by many US ethicists. For example, Veatch and Spicer (1992) maintain that a physician is obliged to supply requested treatment even if the request 'deviates intolerably' from established standards or is in terms of the doctor's judgement 'grossly inappropriate'.

In discussion of this we should note, first, that Veatch and Spicer, and many other US ethicists who hold this view of patient autonomy, are surely mistaken if they think that it follows from any interpretation of the doctrine of autonomy that people should be given something simply on the grounds that they demand it.

Secondly, we must remember that the principle of respect for autonomy applies not only to the patient but to the doctor, and if in the doctor's professional opinion the requested treatment is 'grossly inappropriate', then the doctor has no duty to provide it; indeed he or she has a duty not to provide it. This position has in fact been supported in the UK by the Court of Appeal. In a case in which a physician had indicated that he would not concur with a family's request to give a dying patient ventilatory treatment if that became necessary to sustain the patient's life, Lord Justice Donaldson stated that 'courts should not require a medical practitioner ... to adopt a course of treatment which in the *bona fide* clinical judgement of the practitioner was contraindicated.' Lord Justice Balcome went further and wrote that he 'could conceive of no situation where it would be proper to order a doctor to treat a patient in a manner contrary to his or her clinical judgement'. In other words, the Court of Appeal is here supporting the professional autonomy of the doctor (Re J. 1992).

Thirdly, let us consider the change in ethos or culture which is leading to the consumer view of autonomy, and the implications of the change for the main tradition of the doctor–patient relationship. It will be remembered that in a true consumer situation the shoe salesperson, having advised me against buying shoes which are 'grossly inappropriate' for my purposes, has no duty to refuse the sale if I insist on buying them. What are the implications of importing these consumer assumptions into the doctor–patient relationship?

The most obvious implication is that medicine will cease to be a profession and will become a service industry. If that happens the ethics of medicine will completely change. Indeed, some might argue that the need for ethics of any kind will vanish because the discipline of the market will replace the need for ethics. But we prefer to say that traditional medical ethics (which have grown up to protect the vulnerable patient against exploitation) will be replaced by the ethics of consumerism. And this is indeed being encouraged by the British Government. Let us look briefly at the ethics of consumerism.

Consumer ethics tend to highlight the following concepts. Consumers must have *access* to the services or goods they require; they must have *choice* of the goods or services they require; and this will involve *competition* between suppliers and a fair balance in the market place between supplier and customer; consumers must have *adequate information* on the goods and services they require, and the information must be expressed in clear language; it must be possible for the customer to obtain *redress* in the event of poor services or goods; the products or services must be *safe and subject to regulation* to ensure safety.

A consumer ethic of this kind underlies the idea of the free market and it is certainly appropriate in some areas of life. The question is whether it is appropriate in health care. It has at least two important implications: health care becomes a commodity like any other in the market, and the carers make up a service industry. It is not possible in this short introduction to discuss the far-reaching implications of such a change in ethos or to evaluate it. We shall simply note in summary that one and the same concept of patient autonomy is open to two different interpretations—and in the case of the second interpretation gives rise to a radically different view of medical practice from the traditional one. In Chapter 2 on the carer–patient relationship we explore the implications of these two different interpretations of the concept of patient autonomy for medical practice, and there we argue that the traditional view may have more to offer in terms of health care delivery than the more recent idea of consumer autonomy.

1.5   Utility and justice

Whether or not we adopt the traditional or the consumer view of the doctor–patient relationship, we must come to terms with the need for rationing in health care. Now some people may argue that rationing, while it raises important issues, does not raise ethical issues. The assumption of this position is that ethics has to do only with the face-to-face situation. We believe this view to be inadequate. Questions of the supply and fair distribution of resources are matters of ethics, and the general ethical principles which are relevant are those of utility and justice. Utility is the principle concerned with maximizing outcomes or preferences. In the old formulation it tells us to seek the greatest happiness of the greatest number. As such, the principle of utility says nothing about how the greatest happiness should be distributed; an aggregate of utility A might be greater than an aggregate of B, but we might still give our moral approval to the situation which produces B rather than A, on the grounds that in B the benefits are more fairly distributed. It has been a long-running debate within moral philosophy as to whether our moral judgement for B can still somehow be subsumed under the principle of utility. Without prejudging that debate it might still be clearer to work with two principles rather than with the single principle of utility, because we can then face up to the moral tension between the claims of justice, fairness, or equality, on the one hand, and utility, on the other. This is a debate which is of the first importance to palliative care units (see Chapter 12).

The ethical problems which derive from the tension between equity and utility arise in different areas of health care. One such is the area of distribution. Granted standard services, how ought they to be distributed? If we emphasize the principle of utility, then resources should be concentrated on large centres of population; but this is clearly unfair to those living in rural areas, who would be obliged to travel unreasonable distances for health care.

There a second question of *what* services should be available. Media attention, and indeed medical research interests, are typically directed towards the highly technical end of medicine, such as intensive care units, and because the public imagination is captured by the high-tech services, politicians are sympathetic towards the demands of prominent high-tech consultants. But it is arguable whether this is the best use of scarce health care resources. Greater utility might result from putting the millions into health education, anti-smoking campaigns, and subsidies for fruit and vegetables in urban areas than from heart transplant units. It is obvious that palliative care, which comes at the lower end of the technological spectrum, will be involved in a struggle for resources.

There is a third area in which there can be tensions between utility and justice and that is in the measurement of quality in health care (and indeed elsewhere, such as in the field of education). Utility commits us to evaluating outcomes, to setting targets, to auditing everything that can be audited, and many activities which cannot. Now evaluation programmes, seen in this way under the umbrella of 'utility', require the introduction of scales of measurement, and if there is going to be measurement there must be units of measurement. The consequence of this is that what is not in measurable units tends to be regarded as unimportant. To put it differently, and controversially, quality is interpreted in quantitative terms, and consequently in some areas of health care, where quality is not easily quantifiable, quality is marginalized. For example, how is quality to be measured in the palliative area of health care? As a result of the desire to quantify (which is an implication of utility), there can be injustice in the evaluation of some services, such as palliative care.

A fourth area in which utility and justice can conflict is that of research. Medical research is important to ensure continual improvement in the quality of patient care, and also the good use of scarce resources. Examples abound of such improvements—such as new laser techniques in surgery which are good for patients but also good for scarce resources. Research is therefore an imperative of utility. But the randomized trials and other sorts of intervention involved in research may not be in the best interests of given patients, even though codes of ethics always state that the interests of individual patients must be given priority over every other consideration. Some patients must therefore be unfairly treated in the interests of general utility. We could also describe this as a clash between beneficence or non-maleficence and utility. It is irrelevant to this conflict whether patients have consented or not (although of course their autonomy will also be infringed if they have not). This conflict seems irresolvable, and it is acute in the area of palliation (see Chapter 11).

1.6 Compassion, the virtues, and se ... elopment

We shall conclude with a discussion ... wo areas of health care ethics which have tended to be negle ... but are now being more stressed in nursing literature and inde ... re generally in feminism.

The first neglected aspect of moral ... the self-regarding aspect. Some philosophers deny that there c ... a self-regarding side to morality, for they see morality as ... ng an essentially social function, concerned only with regu ... one's conduct *vis-à-vis* other members of society. Such a vi ... s developed out of one strand in J. S. Mill's thinking. Mill i ... essay *On Liberty* (1859) seemed to be arguing that moral issue ... e only to the extent that one's conduct harms other people; in ... as one's conduct affects only oneself it does not raise a moral ... . Yet in the same work, Mill has a chapter on 'self-developm ... Chapter 3) in which the importance of developing certain pers ... traits is stressed. As he puts it, 'It really is of importance no ... what men do, but also what manner of men they are that do ... nd this view, that there are moral duties to cultivate in onesel ... in characteristic human excellences, goes back to Plato and A ... le and is taken up in a slightly different form by the Judaeo-C ... an traditions. According to these traditions human nature can ' ... sh' and should therefore be cultivated, or we have a duty to cu ... e the talents we have in trust. For Kant, the principle (or attitu ... ich is often stated in the form of 'One ought to respect auton ... s persons' is more fully stated as 'Respect human nature, whe ... your own person or in that of another' (Kant 1785, Chapter 2 ... ther words, Kant makes ample room for the idea of a self-rega ... area of morality.

This is an important area of mor ... for those in the caring professions, and it is the more importa ... that its neglect can seem a virtue. It is quite common for profe ... l carers to live a life of devotion to their patients as a result of ... their own lives become empty and impoverished. They have ... ated only their medical knowledge and skills and have nothin ... y on anything else.

The duty of self-development can a ... justified in terms of its benefits to other people. Since so muc ... the success of a doctor, nurse, dentist, or other health worker ... nds on the relationship each has with a patient, and since th ... re of that relationship depends partly on the patient's percep ... of the helper, it is vital that the professional should be seen a ... authentic human being who happens to be a doctor, nurse, or other carer. There is a moral element in the most technical-seeming medical or nursing judgement. If that is so, then it is important that these judgements should be the products not just of a technical, scientific mind, but of a humane and compassionate one. That is why it is important for the health care professional to be *more* than just that; to be a morally developed person who happens to follow a given professional path. Self-development, then, is good both for its own sake and for what it gives to patients, friends, and families.

It has recently been argued (Pellegrino and Thomasma 1993) that medical ethics stresses principles too much and feelings not enough—that caring, which is said to be a distinctively female virtue, has been neglected. We shall call this moral quality 'compassion', or suffering with someone.

The natural ingredients of compassion are part of the make-up of a normal human being. We all have the capacity to feel with others, to enter to some extent into their predicaments and share their emotions. This capacity is displayed even in an extreme situation, for it is the basis of the strategy for dealing with terrorists who have taken hostages, namely to delay doing anything as long as possible on the grounds that it is emotionally difficult to kill hostages if you have shared experiences with them. This capacity to identify with the feelings of others is the natural basis of compassion.

Compassion, however, is not just a matter of having informed feelings for particular others—it is not just passive. To have compassion is to be moved to act on the basis of the promptings of natural emotion. We prefer the old-fashioned term 'compassion' to the semi-technical term 'empathy' on the grounds that the latter suggests something passive and, indeed, over-professionalized. In a similar way, the term 'sympathy' is ambiguous as between passive and active modes of expression. If someone is described as 'very sympathetic' this might mean simply that he/she shared one's feelings, or that he/she went on to do something about one's predicament. To be compassionate, however, requires both responses.

We are maintaining, then, that true compassion has an *affective* aspect—we feel with others—a *cognitive* aspect—we have particularized insight into the situation of others—and a *conative* aspect—we are moved to act on behalf of others. Compassion cannot ever replace principles, but so understood it provides an essential supplement to them.

Compassion is the virtue most often stressed in health care ethics, but other virtues are also important. For example, courage is important. Courage is most often thought to be the virtue which enables us to act as we ought when we are fearful of physical danger. But other situations can also require courage. Sometimes angry relatives make demands which are unreasonable or might not be in the best interests of the patient, and threaten legal action unless their demands are met. It takes courage to face up to relatives in such situations and explain why their demands cannot be granted. We shall discuss this further in our chapter on dealing with relatives. Courage may also be required when dealing with senior colleagues or management, if they are pursuing policies not in the best interests of patients. Palliative care is sometimes regarded as less important than curative or life-prolonging treatments and courage may be required to query at management meetings whether, for instance, chemotherapy should take so much of the budget that insufficient is left for palliative care of terminally ill patients.

It is well known that health carers lead busy lives. Now busyness is not simply a matter of long hours; it can also mean several demands being made on one's attention at the same time. Or it can mean conflicting demands, or demands of different sorts being made at the same time. For example, there may be a need to give teaching to a less than reliable junior, while conscious that an angry or distressed relative is waiting to be interviewed and a very sick patient urgently needs a change of medication. The virtue which is needed in such situations of stress is equanimity, the disposition to stay calm and deal competently and firmly but politely with each problem. All without raising one's blood pressure.

In sum, we are arguing that the practice of health care ethics requires a framework of principles. The two most ancient principles—of non-maleficence and beneficence—are nowadays supplemented by another two—of respect for the patient's autonomous decisions, and of justice. All four ought to govern our face-to-face encounters with patients. But nowadays doctors and nurses face problems of rationing. If these problems are to be solved in an ethical manner, then the principle of justice must be extended beyond the face-to-face encounter and be applied to society; we must not only treat *this* patient fairly but also distribute resources fairly among *all* patients. Moreover, we must make the most efficient use of resources, and therefore we must add the fifth principle of utility.

These five principles govern our relationships with others, but we must also add a sixth principle and respect human nature in our own person.

Whereas some writers give greater emphasis to some of these principles—such as respecting autonomy or maximizing utility—we do not. We freely admit that the principles will sometimes conflict, and when that happens what is needed is what Aristotle called *phronesis* or practical wisdom, a concept we shall explain in the next section. Principles provide the framework, but we must remember our feelings; the morally good person is not just principled, but also compassionate.

1.7   The aims of palliative care: personal, intrinsic, and extrinsic

> *Every art and every investigation, and likewise every practical pursuit or undertaking, seems to aim at some good: hence it has been said that the good is that at which all things aim.*
>
> Aristotle, *Nicomachean Ethics*, Bk 1

Palliative care is not an 'island' of philosophy and practice for a few privileged patients and staff. It is an integral part of effective health care. Its aims and scope should therefore fall within those of health care, and its philosophy must be compatible with that of a comprehensive health service, whether publicly or privately funded. In clarifying the aims of palliative care we shall consequently relate them as appropriate to the aims of health care more generally. In particular, we shall express the aims of palliative care in terms of distinctions and concepts which are applicable to any area of health care.

In any discussion of the aims of health care it is common to find those who give it a narrow focus—say, one concerned with treating disease processes—and those who give it a wide focus—say, one which would include the total mental and social well-being of the patient and perhaps the relatives as well. In the course of such discussion it is usually admitted that professionals also have personal aims (not least of which is earning a living!). What is needed here is the drawing of some distinctions (Downie and Charlton 1992).

In the first place, a person who happens to be a doctor or nurse will have various aims which are not necessarily connected with health care although they are furthered by it. Let us call these 'personal aims'. For example, a doctor or nurse might aim at earning a living, at having job security, or at expressing idealism. These are legitimately regarded as among their aims by the doctor or nurse in that they fulfil them by means of their occupations. But they are not connected with health care as such, since they might just as easily be satisfied by other occupations. Hence they can be identified as 'personal aims'. Note that it does not follow from the fact that they are not connected with health care as such that they are un-important. Indeed, it may be that job satisfaction or dissatisfaction are in fact largely connected with the opportunities of the doctor or nurse to fulfil personal aims through the practice of health care. This is especially true in the field of palliative care.

Secondly, and most importantly, there is what we shall call the 'intrinsic aim' of health care, the aim which must be entertained by anyone practising any form of health care. We shall maintain that in palliative care, as in the rest of health care, the intrinsic aim is to bring about what we shall call a 'medical good'. The term 'medical good' can never be precisely or completely analysed but we are using it as a blanket term to cover medical treatments such as those which lead to the amelioration or sometimes cure of disease processes, the relief of suffering, the prolongation of life, the dressing of wounds or injuries, and many others. It is a characteristic feature of the treatments which lead to this 'medical good' that they are brought about by the use of drugs or technical procedures. It hardly needs to be said, but we stress it, that such treatments would not succeed unless they were delivered in a context of dedicated nursing care. In other words, to assert that the intrinsic aim of all health care is to bring about a medical good, so understood, is not in any way to suggest that the role of other team members is less important than that of doctors, or that patients do not require caring as much as treatment in order to attain their medical good.

Nevertheless, it will be objected by many working in palliative care, and perhaps also in other areas of health care, that we have wrongly accepted too narrow a focus for the aim of health care. The patient's good, it will be said, is more than simply the patient's medical good. In palliative care, for example, the carers need to cope with the emotional problems of the patient and the family, not to mention with their spiritual anxieties. Dealing with such matters involves dealing with what is wider than is reasonably called a 'medical good'.

To reply to this important kind of objection we require to introduce another category of aim for health care. We shall call this the 'extrinsic' aim. To ask about the extrinsic aim of palliative care is to ask about what doctors and nurses may be able to do as a result of standing in the special relationships with their patients (see Chapter 2) which is the condition of fulfilling the intrinsic aim. In their attempt to fulfil their intrinsic aim of bringing about a medical good, doctors and nurses may gain insights into the background anxieties and fears of patients, and because of their special relationship they may sometimes be in a position to do something about these fears and worries. The provision of this kind of service we shall call the 'extrinsic' aim of health care. It is clearly an aim of health care because it is connected with a medical good such as the relief of suffering. We can call it the promotion of the patient's psychological good (using the term 'psychological' in a very broad way to cover emotional, relational, and spiritual goods). But why do we call the promotion of this psychological good an 'extrinsic' aim?

The first reason is because in pursuing this aim doctors and nurses are attempting to alleviate conditions which constitute the psychological or social backgrounds to, or the emotional consequences of, the patient's primary problems rather than the medical problems themselves. Secondly, and more importantly, there are no skills which professionally qualify a carer for dealing with these resultant states. Anything which is correctly called a professional expertise must have a knowledge base, and there is no body of expert knowledge which can deal with the range and complexity of people's emotional, relational, or social problems. There is clearly an expertise for furthering the medical good which it is the primary aim of health care to promote. But there is very little professional expertise for dealing with the rest. Patients are likely to be anxious, distressed, depressed, and perhaps angry and aggressive. No doubt some knowledge of the relevant social sciences will provide a helpful background to dealing with such problems, and no doubt some of them are treatable, and are in fact treated, as medical problems. But is it appropriate to medicalize all aspects of human experience? Does palliative or any kind of health care mean that painful emotions, loneliness, guilt, and anxiety should all be extinguished by the right sort of drug treatment, or by a learned stereotyped response on behalf of the professional?

Some people may argue that while it is inappropriate to medicalize every human problem, there are other professional skills—counselling skills, for example—which can provide the professional supplement to medical and nursing skills. Together, the medical skills, nursing skills, and counselling skills can comprise a total professional approach which can deal with any emotional or relational problem. This is an illusion. For any truly professional expertise there must exist a shared and learned knowledge base and there is no such knowledge base which can supply professional skills for dealing with normal human emotions. Hence we call the pursuit of this broadly psychological good of the patient an extrinsic aim of health care.

We wish to claim, then, that palliative care, like other forms of health care, has two radically different types of component. First, there are the professional skills which derive from the knowledge bases of medicine, nursing, social work, and allied health care professions. The exercise of these skills constitutes the primary or intrinsic aim of palliative care and it is aimed at what we have termed the 'medical good' of the patient. But sometimes the patient may bring up problems and worries concerned with their relationship with a spouse or parent, or regrets about their present or past life. Are we suggesting that the team should ignore these psychological problems? Not exactly. Dealing with them, in so far as they can be dealt with at all, is part of what we call the extrinsic aim of palliative care. As a consequence of wide experience of palliative care, and life in general, and influenced by their own personality, the members of a team may develop practical wisdom to assist with a range of human issues. This constitutes the second component of palliative care.

How are we to describe this second component, and how can it be acquired? It was described by Aristotle as *phronesis* or practical wisdom, and it is an ability we all have to some extent. It can be cultivated through wide experience of life, but it can never be a professional expertise produced by going on a course. At a seminar on 'Helping Bereaved Parents' it was said that the person best at it in that particular section of the paediatric hospital was not the counsellor, clergyman, or psychiatrist; it was the ward maid. She was not likely to have had advanced education, or to have attended courses, but she was likely to have had a rich experience of life. Her *phronesis* or practical wisdom was derived from the impact of this experience on her unique personality.

It is true of course that the pursuit of their intrinsic aim may help carers to acquire the experience of life which will assist them in dealing with the wider issues which constitute their extrinsic aim. But we do not gain all of our practical wisdom from our professional roles; much of it must come from our experience of life outside the job. Ordinary life experience is often undervalued in this respect. For instance, our relationships inside the workplace are insufficiently close to give us understanding of very close, loving relationships. We have to experience these in our own personal lives outside the workplace in order to give us some knowledge of such relationships so that we may have some ability to understand the loving relationships of our patients. There is no professional training that enables us to achieve this sort of understanding which forms the base of our wider or extrinsic aim (see also Chapter 10).

From one point of view, then, we are insisting on this distinction between intrinsic and extrinsic aims to prevent the concept of palliative care becoming so wide that no training would qualify a person to undertake it, and no treatment could count as adequate. Indeed, palliative care must be undertaken by all doctors and nurses, albeit to a variable extent. All must be capable of basic competence in the care of those terminally ill. In order for this to be possible as an aim for all involved in health care, the knowledge and skills required must be such that they can be acquired by training. This can be true only for care and treatment needed to remove or alleviate physical suffering and mental illness. Thus only the intrinsic aim of palliative care can be considered a goal and reasonable aim for all health care professionals. We can all be trained to aim at a medical good. On the other hand, our abilities in dealing with psychological, emotional, and spiritual distress will always vary as our understanding, which is derived from our own personalities and life experiences, will vary. Hence, from this point of view the pursuit of the patient's psychological good through the exercise of the carer's *phronesis* or practical wisdom counts as the extrinsic aim.

But there is another point of view from which we can look at the exercise of the technical skills which advance the intrinsic aim or medical good and the exercise of the practical wisdom which advances the extrinsic aim of psychological good. From this second point of view it is practical wisdom which is the dominant or controlling element in care. This theme will recur in various contexts. As professional expertise develops it is easy to assume that there can be an algorithm for every problem, that ideally decisions can be reached by following the relevant guidelines or flow charts. This is a dangerous illusion. Science and social science can tell us only (although it is crucially important) what is for the most part so: practical wisdom tells us what in this particular case is so. Hence, it must be the controlling element in any kind of care. Professional knowledge and skills suggest the range of possible treatments: practical wisdom leads to a judgement as to which of these is appropriate in a given case in the light of many factors, including the meaning of the disease and the treatment for the patient. Moreover, and this is an additional point, practical wisdom also suggests the *manner* in which treatment should be given or information given. For example, we shall later (Chapter 6) discuss the imparting of information. It will emerge that the manner of giving it may be just as important as its content. Humane treatment flows from the carer with practical wisdom.

From this second point of view practical wisdom is the central concept in palliative care or indeed in all health care. The techniques through which the medical good can be pursued do not of themselves tell us when, to what extent, or in what manner, they ought to be pursued. Techniques are blind and require the guidance of the ethical concept of practical wisdom. Moreover, by making practical wisdom the controlling element in the pursuit of both the medical good and the psychological good of the patient, we have avoided compartmentalizing the two aims. Both must be controlled by the underlying ethical concern of practical wisdom, which is therefore the controlling moral component in all palliative care.

1.8 Whole person care

> *Life is short, science is long; opportunity is elusive, experience is dangerous, judgement is difficult. It is not enough for the physician to do what is necessary, but the patient and the attendants must do their part as well, and circumstances must be favourable.*
>
> *Hippocrates, from Aphorisms*

Our strategy has been to introduce the conceptual distinctions between personal aims, intrinsic aims, and extrinsic aims so that we may have a framework in which to examine one of the central ideas in the specialty of palliative care—whole person or holistic care[1] or care aimed not just at a medical good or a psychological good, but at the patient's total good, or best interests.

Wholeness, or overall well-being, is often said to be the ultimate goal of human life. Clearly, many things can go wrong as we all pursue this goal. Important among these mishaps is the occurrence of diseases and illnesses. Hence the health care professions have come into existence to remove or help us over these particular obstacles, and to care for our suffering when we stumble on them. This was the justification for making a medical good such as the relief of suffering the intrinsic aim of all health care. But clearly there are many more impediments to the pursuit of wholeness—such as emotional or spiritual distress, social isolation, financial difficulties, and so on. For some of these problems there exists at best a limited expertise. For example, the clergy may be able to soothe the troubled spirit and social workers may be able to assist with damp housing. But the limitation on professional expertise in dealing with these matters was the main reason we have so far given for describing the attempts by health carers to grapple with such obstacles to wholeness as an extrinsic aim of health care.

There is, however, another reason for advising caution, or modesty, before claiming that in palliative or any kind of health care we can aim at treating the whole person. The reason is stated in Shakespeare's *Macbeth* (Act V, Scene 3).

> *Macbeth:* *Canst thou not minister to a mind diseased,*
> *Pluck from the memory a rooted sorrow,*
> *Raze out the written troubles of the brain,*
> *And with some sweet oblivious antidote*
> *Cleanse the stuff'd bosom of that perilous stuff*
> *Which weighs upon the heart?*
> *Doctor:* *Therein the patient*
> *Must minister to himself.*

In other words, Shakespeare is saying that we cannot make any helpful impact on the psychological, social, or spiritual condition of another, unless the subject is actively involved. The subjects cannot be passive in this process—if they are the attempt is bound to be ineffective. In contrast, physical illness can be influenced by external factors such as drugs or technological interventions without much active participation by the patient. That is why we regard the provision of such care as the intrinsic aim of all health care and the primary responsibility of the health care professional.

The palliative care team cannot bear the sole responsibility for the psychological, social, and spiritual well-being of the patient, because it can influence those states only in partnership with the patient. A partnership implies that both are actively involved. The team cannot bear responsibility for something over which they have very little control. The patient (unless mentally ill) has by far the most control over his or her own psychological good.

It might be said that even if carers have little control over the emotional state of a patient, they can at least try to understand that state. Sometimes this kind of understanding is called 'empathy'. Now no doubt some carers can sometimes achieve this with some patients, but the belief that we can be trained to empathize is a dangerous illusion. It is hard enough to understand someone with whom one has lived for twenty years; the possibility of understanding a patient is therefore remote. But just as it is possible to love completely without complete understanding, so it is possible to give humane treatment without complete emotional understanding. The important point is that we must respect the patient as an individual unique among others. It is this moral imperative of practical wisdom which qualifies the pursuit of both the intrinsic and the extrinsic aim of palliative care. It follows that it must also underlie the concept of whole person care.

Paradoxically, it is precisely the fact that whole person care implies respect for the patient's own personal goals and values that imposes limits on the scope of professional activity directed towards such care. We must not attempt to inflict unwanted attention or solutions to emotional or social problems on the patient, any more than we would inflict unwanted physical treatment without the patient's informed consent. Recognition of this limitation is an integral part of the concept of whole person care, because included in this concept is the control individuals always have over their own psychological, social, and spiritual well-being. Thus we must accept that no treatment or care can be given which the informed and competent patient does not want. This is a necessity of practical wisdom which is recognized in terms of consent to physical treatment, but is sometimes regarded with less respect in terms of psychological care. But recognition of the limits to psychological care must be underlined because it acts as a safeguard against the setting of unrealistic goals for the patient and the team. Respect for the patient's wishes in all forms of care is an ethical necessity; it is integral to the concept of whole person care.

Whole person care implies responsibility for influencing physical and mental illness states and minimizing distress from them, in partnership with the patient. It also implies a willingness to assist the patient to overcome psychological, social, and spiritual barriers to well-being, by using our relationship with them as fellow members of a community. In this last task we are acting not so much in our professional roles but more as a caring companion who has had the benefit of listening to the experiences and feelings of many previous patients in similar situations.

It is a by-product of this aspect of palliative care that patients tend to feel that their worth as individuals has been affirmed, both by society which continues to manifest care for them by expending resources on them when they are dying, and also by any person in the health care team who treats them competently and compassio-nately and with respect for their preferences and values. It is in this way that palliative care affirms the value of each patient, even when physical and mental function is much less than optimal and may be irreversibly declining.

We therefore give a cautious acceptance to the concept of whole person or holistic care. It can encapsulate the intrinsic aim of palliative care—the medical good such as the relief of suffering—and also the extrinsic aim—the offer of help for emotional, spiritual, or relational problems. We must repeat once again, however, that the extrinsic aim is not mainly based on professional expertise, but on the practical wisdom of a compassionate and experienced human being, and that the help can only be offered; if it is to succeed at all it can only be in partnership with the patient. It might in fact be less misleading to speak of the 'humane' carer rather than the 'holistic' carer, but the term 'holistic' is endemic in palliative care literature. Hence, we shall use it, but with caution, for it may be both misleading and pretentious. The safeguard is to remember the ethical rule of practical wisdom that we ought to respect the values of other unique individuals. Their values, or their total good or well-being as they perceive it, may not correspond to their medical good as seen by the team.

1.9 Relatives

Similar considerations arise as to whether the relatives as well as the patient are part of the remit of palliative care. It seems to us that to include the care of relatives within the intrinsic aim of palliative care is unrealistic; resources are stretched enough in doing a reasonable job caring for patients and considering their interests. Conflicts of interests between the needs of the patient and those of the relatives, both in terms of treatment preferences and allocation of the valuable resource of professional time, are inevitable if the care of relatives is seen as part of the intrinsic aim of palliative care.

Moreover, and this is a second point, if the reason for including relatives and friends within the remit of the team is that they are anxious, distressed, or sad, as the relatives of dying patients may well be, this amounts to an attempt to medicalize ordinary human experience. This implies that dealing with such experience and emotional reactions to it requires a certain professional expertise. In fact, anxiety, grief, loneliness, and general unhappiness are the lot of all of us at certain times in life; they are not conditions re-quiring professional treatment. And the idea that there are special professional skills, counselling skills, which are appropriate for grieving relatives because they can in some way alleviate that grief, is a delusion. Of course, as we have said, palliative care also has what we have called 'extrinsic' aims. As a result of experience in caring for patients, the doctors, nurses, and others concerned are exposed to painful situations and must make difficult decisions. These experiences, plus those of life in general, can generate a humane practical wisdom, and it is a reasonable extrinsic aim of palliative care to pass on this wisdom to patients and relatives. We shall discuss the issues of dealing with relatives in Chapter 3.

1.10 Ethics and aims

We are now in a position to bring together both main themes of the chapter and to make explicit the way in which the ethical concepts and principles of the first theme are integrated with the aims of the second theme. We would argue that the aims of palliative care themselves give rise to the principles which have been described in Section 1.4 as beneficence, non-maleficence, respect for autonomy,

pment. The intrinsic aim of palliative
medical good such as the relief of
ngs from the principle of beneficence,
lp, which must go *in tandem* with the
)f not harming the patient, in order
:atment do not outweigh its benefits.
alify the pursuit of the extrinsic aims
principle—the need to respect the
an important safeguard against
.... interventions undertaken in pursuit of either the intrinsic
or the extrinsic aims. Indeed, it is not logically possible to further the
extrinsic aim of the patient's psychological good unless that patient's
own goals, values, and choices are respected. At the same time, that
principle reminds us that the professional's autonomy is also to be
respected. Finally, the pursuit of the intrinsic and extrinsic aims of
palliative care for a patient population requires health care professionals to act justly by distributing the benefits of that care fairly,
and also to maximize the overall benefits of that care.

Nevertheless, whilst clear concepts of the aims of palliative care
and the ethical principles which govern its practice are *necessary* for
health care professionals, they are not *sufficient* to ensure that each
individual patient receives the care most appropriate to his or her
unique needs, and that such care is selected and delivered in a
humane and compassionate manner. In a sense we might say that
the aims and ethical principles of palliative care form part of its
'science', which is about generalities, whereas the 'art' of palliative
care, which is about particularities, lies in finding the best course of
action for each unique patient. The science gives us general aims and
principles, but the art is essential in applying them to reach the best
solution in each unique clinical situation. Moreover, the art of
palliative care must not be lost in the pursuit of its science.

How can we further characterize the art of palliative care? First, in
Section 1.6 we spoke of virtues and dispositions as well as principles.
It matters to patients that their carers have warm and compassionate
dispositions. This was the ethical point behind our preference for the
concept of the 'humane' carer, doctor or nurse, rather than the
'holistic' carer. As we have stressed, 'holistic' care can be carried out
in an inconsiderate or inhumane manner, and equally the most
physical of treatments can be carried out in a humane manner. The
important point is that whether it is the intrinsic or the extrinsic aim

which is being furthered, its pursuit must be in a compassionate and humane manner. Secondly, in Section 1.7 we stressed the importance of *phronesis*, or practical wisdom, as the controlling moral component of palliative care. Such wisdom is the pursuit of the best ends by the best means (Hutcheson 1725) in the clinical situation. Thus the virtues of compassion and practical wisdom are essential to the art of palliative care. Any patient can tell the difference between someone who is a genuinely compassionate and caring human being, and someone who simply gives wooden or stereotyped responses.

But how are professional carers to develop these virtues? Not by going on courses! As we shall discuss later (Chapter 10) in more detail, it makes no sense to speak of courses in genuineness or wisdom! Perhaps in the end some people, by nature or God's grace, just are wise, caring, and compassionate and others are not. But two points are worth making in practical qualification of this conclusion.

The first requires us to remember that at the beginning of Section 1.7 we identified what we called the 'personal' aims of the health care professional. They are the aims which the carer may fulfil via the job, although they are not directly related to the job in that they may be fulfilled in other jobs. Many doctors and nurses express their idealism through their work in palliative care. Some of those working in the specialty have strong religious commitments and feel they have a mission to care for the dying. In so far as personal aims can be fulfilled through the exercise of a profession, job-satisfaction will result, and it will be to that extent easier for the doctor or nurse to be genuinely compassionate. Strong religious convictions also give meaning to life and sustain professional carers who continuously confront death and loss. It must also be remembered, however, that there can be a pathological side to deeply held personal aims, especially the religious ones. This is the pathology of the 'hidden agenda', and it is one we warned against when discussing the limitations and dangers of overenthusiastic pursuit of the extrinsic aim of palliative care. The dying patient is highly vulnerable to those who believe they have the truth about life and death.

The second point relates to the carer's ability to sustain the mentally and emotionally tiring struggle of continuous attempts to attain and maintain the virtues of compassion and practical wisdom amidst the pressures of health care. All too often the carer becomes emotionally exhausted, or 'burnt out'. Quite simply, they have passed into a state of 'negative emotional balance', caused by too

much emotional output insufficiently replenished by input. It constitutes a harm which cannot be sustained indefinitely.

Antidotes to this pathological process are provided by interests
and relationships outside the job. Such interests give perspective to
the life of professional care and prevent obsessions taking root.
These interests may be family ones, or sporting ones, or artistic ones,
but the important point is that whatever they are they must provide
broader horizons. Close personal relationships outside the workplace sustain professional carers, as well as increasing their ability
to understand the relationships of those they care for. Interests and
relationships provide a sustaining and enriching broad experience
of life.

The cultivation of compassion and practical wisdom is not a
matter of moral indifference. We have already argued (p. 13) that
there is a self-referring side to morality. It is a moral duty to cultivate
all the talents we have, and they are likely to be much broader than
those used in our professional duties. Many professionals working in
health care see themselves as involved in a life of dedication; they
give themselves for others. Yes, but they should ask themselves what
they have to give, and what is to sustain them in the giving.

1.11 Conclusions

1. In this chapter we have introduced the main concepts which
   are involved in the discussion of the ethical issues of health
   care and we have drawn attention to the way in which what
   we have called the 'main tradition' of medical ethics has been
   broadened and is now more appropriately called the tradition
   of 'health care' ethics.

2. The intrinsic aim of palliative care, as part of health care, is
   the promotion of a medical good related to physical or mental
   illness.

3. This professional treatment must be humane and show full
   appreciation of the meaning of the disease, suffering, and
   treatment for the particular patient, or of its place in the
   patient's conception of his total good.

4. Palliative care also has extrinsic aims. As a result of their
   professional experience those involved in palliation may be

able to offer a range of advice and discussion based on practical wisdom generated by interaction between their own personality and their experience of health care and life in general.

5. What is called 'whole person' or 'holistic' care is an amalgam of care deriving from the intrinsic and, where applicable, the extrinsic aim of palliative care. It requires the consent of the patient and can be promoted, if at all, only in partnership with the patient. Only patients can know their own total good.

6. Coping with the problems of relatives is part of the extrinsic rather than the intrinsic aim of palliative care.

7. The ethical concepts introduced are integral to the pursuit of the aims and the controlling virtue is that of practical wisdom. Only the exercise of practical wisdom can ensure that the *carer's* conception of the patient's medical or psychological good is not forced on the patient, whose perceived total good may just be to be left in peace.

Notes

1. The form 'holistic' is older, the 'wh' form appearing first in the fifteenth century. The noun 'holism' was revived in 1926 by J. C. Smuts. He wrote about the tendency of nature to produce wholes from ordered groupings of units.

2

The patient–carer relationship

(Dr Lydgate) ... was an emotional creature, with a flesh-and-blood sense of fellowship which withstood all the abstractions of special study. He cared not only for 'cases', but for John and Elizabeth, especially Elizabeth.

George Eliot, *Middlemarch*, Ch. XV (1871)

All palliative care is ultimately delivered through the common pathway of the patient–carer relationship. Therefore, the success of such care is dependent on the nature of that relationship, which forms the basis of the practice of health care. Discussions about the nature of such a relationship must be grounded in a clear concept of its purpose.

What sort of patient–carer relationship would be appropriate to meet the aims of palliative care as discussed in Chapter 1? What are the special circumstances of the patient–carer contact in palliative care? In addressing these questions it is helpful to consider the ways in which we use the term 'relationship' in everyday language. It is used in two ways: to stand for the bond which links two or more people, or to stand for the attitudes which bonded people have for each other. The first is a way of describing the role link between people, such as teacher–pupil, and the second is about the attitudes which bonded or linked people have for each other, such as fear, respect, or love.

The two kinds of relationship are connected in complex ways. For example, the teacher–pupil bond is via a role link, but the attitude that teacher and pupil have for each other can vary greatly between respect, love, fear, and so on. It is a matter of opinion which combination of attitudes is most conducive to achieving the educational aim of this relationship, and fortunately it is not necessary to consider it further here! Our task is to discuss the patient–carer relationship and we shall consider both the nature of the role link and the appropriateness of various attitudes.

It is important to emphasize that the study of a role link is about finding the patterns or similarities in the ways patients and carers interact. It is about how people tend to behave when they become patients, and how people tend to behave when they become carers. As in the social sciences, it is to do with discovering patterns or similarities in the way people are and act when in different roles. The ensuing discussion is not about a particular doctor–patient or nurse–patient relationship, for we all know that each and every contact between two people is unique, and that no individual is fixed in their role. Rather it is about the generalities of carer–patient contacts, and about what we can learn and deduce from these generalities which may help us to derive ideas about appropriate attitudes, values, and behaviour in the context of the relationship. Consideration of the moral issues in the relationship is about how people should think, feel, and act as patients or carers.

2.1 The patient's aims in the relationship

What does the patient want from the carer? Sometimes in situations of great physical or emotional distress patients may not have a clearly formulated idea of their desires and expectations. However, they do have a general idea of the desired outcome and this will depend on their personal values and priorities. This idea of the desired outcome, that which they feel will contribute most to their overall well-being or wholeness, is what we have termed their view of their 'total good' or best interests. It is a deeply personal concept which some find difficult to articulate. The patient's idea of their 'total good' is fundamentally known only to them, although others who know them well may have an opinion about it. It is derived from the combination of their own values and preferences, life plans and social circumstances, together with the limitations their illness is imposing on their physical and mental state. The patient usually also has a concept of bodily good, or 'medical good', which is derived from their illness state and their perceived physical needs. The total good (or best interests) of the patient is therefore derived from the combination of their medical or biological good together with their own beliefs, values, and goals. The carers have knowledge of medical good, and the patient has knowledge of personal goals and values.

Whilst they have an idea of their 'total good', patients quite rightly present with those problems for which they want assistance from the carers, and for which they hope the carers may be able to provide at least partial solutions. This may entail physical care, relief of specific symptoms, or sometimes prolongation of life, which are all commonly understood as intrinsic aims in palliative care. Since the concept of whole person care has become more widely accepted, some will also want help with emotional, social, and other problems which fall within the extrinsic aims of palliative care, and similarly they may want additional help for their families.

It must be noted that the patients' dependency on the carers for these 'goods' causes patients to occupy a position of great vulnerability in relation to carers in the palliative care situation.

2.2   The carer's aim in the relationship

Since the carers provide the service and often also asses its success they have a great deal of control over the nature of care provided. The process of clinical audit, carried out by carers themselves, involves continuous reassessment and alteration of the service towards an ideal which is itself established by the carers. In this way the carers have until recently determined the nature of the service provided. This state of affairs is now changing as constraints of finance and policy are increasingly imposed by the purchasers of palliative care. It seems likely that in the future the purchasers will determine the nature of the service via contracts 'negotiated' with the providers of palliative care, the doctors, nurses, and members of allied professions who in these negotiations are largely represented by managers. Be all this as it may, it is clear that the patients have very little power to influence the nature of care provided. The carers are much more able to determine the service available to patients in general, and so have a high degree of autonomy as a professional community.

The professional involved in palliative care is also likely to be highly motivated to act for the patient's good. It is part of our nature as human beings to be benevolent towards others, especially the vulnerable, and we intuitively regard benevolent acts with approval.

What does the carer seek to achieve from the contact with the patient? This is really a fundamental question about the role of carer, whether doctor, nurse, or allied professional. It is consequently a fundamental question about what it is to be a doctor, nurse, or other carer.

We are proposing that the aim of the carer should accord with that of palliative care. Now, the good which is apparent to the caring team is a 'medical good', but the patient knows what treatments or outcomes are in accord with his or her own goals and values. The management of the patient's problems by the carer is directed towards the pursuit of the medical good as modified by the patient's own goals and values. We believe that this is entailed by the principle of beneficence, which is intrinsic to the practice of palliative care and to the role of carer. For example, one might agree to give chemotherapy to a mother with children who wants to undergo treatment which carries only a small chance of prolonging life and is associated with side-effects, especially if one of her own daughters is terminally ill and she wants to outlive that child. On the other hand, one might not agree to give the same treatment to a patient in similar medical circumstances but less extreme social circumstances. We acknowledge that we must all work within certain constraints, not least of which are the limits of resources and clinical and managerial guidelines which together may restrict the clinical options for care and treatment. However, the final choice of care is determined from the available options by consideration of the patient's perception of total good combined with the medical facts of the particular clinical situation. If the patient's views cannot be known (for instance because the patient is either unable to make choices based on his or her personal values or is unable to communicate) then the choice of care is determined by his or her medical good.

We suggest that this simplified approach clarifies the aim of the carer, which must logically be grounded in the aim of palliative care itself. Clarifying the aim of the carer in the context of the patient–carer relationship enables us to determine the morally appropriate attitudes of the carer to the patient. Such attitudes are those which lead to acts which fulfil the ends of the relationship, namely that of furthering the patient's total good. This approach avoids unresolvable conflicts of role for the carer.

The special circumstances of both the patient and carer have now been described, together with the aims that they each have for the relationship. It is important to note that both the patient and carer should share this same aim for their relationship, namely furthering the patient's overall well-being. If patient and carer do not share this aim, or have other conflicting professional or personal aims, the success of their relationship in benefiting the patient will be seriously compromised. As we have mentioned, it is unfortunately the carer who is more likely to have such competing professional and personal aims. Given that this is unavoidable to some extent, it is important that those other aims remain subordinate to that of the patient's total good.

It is also relevant to this discussion that the patient is pursuing only personal aims in the relationship, whereas the carer is acting in accordance with professional aims. The carer is faced with the more difficult task of reconciling personal and professional aims where these may conflict. For example, the carer may wish to leave work on time to meet a social engagement, but the patient may want to have a fairly prolonged discussion. This creates added difficulties for the carer, and raises the possibility in the patient's mind that the carer may have what may be termed 'conflicts of interest'.

We have concluded that the patient's position is likely to be one of vulnerability together with compromised autonomy, whilst that of the carer is one of power and substantial autonomy. Despite these differences they share the mutual aim. Given their different characteristics, how do they stand in relation to each other, and what is the nature of the bond which is most appropriate? What attitudes should they have to each other in order to achieve their mutual aim? How does society try to ensure that the patient's good is achieved, given the inequalities of power in the relationship?

2.3 'Relativity' in the carer–patient encounter

Further consideration of how the patient and carer stand in relation to each other in palliative care, given their role characteristics, reveals that the most striking feature of their mutual positions is inequality of power.

The most obvious source of this inequality lies firstly in a difference of *knowledge*. The doctor or nurse will always know more about the illness and treatment than the patient. As a frustrated patient once said when an earnest doctor was trying to persuade the patient to make her own decision, 'But doctor, you will always have more information than I have!'

Secondly, it is the carer who decides what *information* the patient should be given about the illness. They determine what should be communicated. The patient's understanding of the nature of the illness, its course and likely prognosis, depends entirely on what the caring team choose to reveal. The patient is totally vulnerable to the carer in this respect. Whilst we would all agree that patients should be told the truth, how much of the truth they should be told is a matter of moral judgement. For example, if a patient asks about the likely outcome of stomach cancer with liver metastases, how many of us would feel it appropriate to tell him that there is a small chance that he may bleed to death during a major haematemesis? Information is necessary to make life plans. For example, a patient cannot make realistic life plans if he thinks he is going to live six months when in fact the likelihood is that he will live only six weeks. Moreover, a patient's understanding regarding treatment is determined by the way information is given. For example, a patient may be told a certain chemotherapy is 'the best' for his or her condition, but this is only information about the comparative benefits of different chemotherapy regimes—it does not inform the patient about the comparison in outcomes between chemotherapy and supportive treatment only.

Patients need information not just in order to choose treatment options but also to make plans for their remaining life. Without such information future planning is impossible. An integral part of the concept of autonomy is the ability to make choices and plans—this has sometimes been described as self-determination. However, this is not possible if the patient is not given relevant information. Thus the carer, in being in control of the relevant knowledge, is also largely in control of the patient's ability to make autonomous life plans.

Thirdly, carers decide what treatment or care *options* should be offered. It is naive to assume that all conceivable treatments could or should be offered to all patients in palliative care. Few people would suggest that doctors should offer treatments they consider definitely futile or harmful (despite a possible interpretation of the Patient's Charter to this effect). Treatments may not be offered because they are not available due to resource constraints, or because they lie outside professional guidelines, because the evidence suggests that their associated harms and risks exceed their benefits. Later we shall discuss how far this limitation and selection of treatment options is justified in particular circumstances. For now it is sufficient to acknowledge that selection of treatment options offered by carers does occur, and it places them in a position of considerable power. It a patient does not know that a certain treatment is possible, they are not in a position to ask for it.

Fourthly, the carer is also in possession of the *skills* which the patient needs, and without which their good cannot be served. This also creates an insuperable difference in the power balance between carer and patient.

Fifthly, the carer, as gatekeeper of *resources*, also has the power to influence the care available to a particular patient; the patient has access to those needed resources only through the carer.

Sixthly, the carer has ultimate control not only of what care is offered and given, but of how such care is given. In other words, the *manner* in which care is delivered is controlled by the carer. For example, an intravenous infusion and a bed-bath can both be given either with gentleness and cheerfulness or in a brusque and rough manner. This aspect of the nature of care lies in the control of the professional, not the patient.

Seventhly, in a social context, the professional may often be more articulate than the patient, who may also be relatively socially disadvantaged. This can create feelings of inferiority in the patient, who may then become disempowered by such feelings. Doctors often have more highly developed *powers of argument* than patients. Thus in a discussion it is more likely that the carer will be able to persuade the patient of the wisdom of his point of view than vice versa.

Eighthly, all the above inequalities are compounded by the fact that many carer–patient contacts occur *not on the patient's home ground* but in a general practitioner's surgery, a hospital clinic, or in a specialist palliative care unit. Moreover, the patient is extremely likely to be outnumbered in these circumstances by a band of knowledgeable professionals united behind a particular point of view.

Ninthly, the carer is likely to be physically fit which means that they are able to stand or sit at will and also to walk away. The *patient may be so frail* that she is necessarily recumbent, and even if able to sit, she is frequently unable to walk away. Whilst the carer can terminate an interview, it is much more difficult for the patient to do so. We are all taught in communication lessons that we should aim to be at the same physical level as the patient, and we know from everyday experience that conversation is easier when this so. Sometimes we go to great lengths to achieve this, often squatting beside a chair or wheelchair if there is nowhere for us to sit, resulting in the rather humorously termed 'compassion crouch'. However, there is no getting away from the fact that we can alter position and in particular can walk away when the patient cannot.

Tenthly, apart from questions of physical position, the question of *strength and stamina* also creates inequalities in the relationship. Whilst the carer can cope with a lengthy conversation about care choices, the lethargic, exhausted, or nauseated patient is completely unable to, and there is a danger of the patient agreeing quickly in order to terminate an interview which they find unendurable because of the effort of sustaining concentration and conversation. The patient may take the path of least resistance and agree with the carer's suggestions. There is no easy solution to this problem if we are going to encourage patients to participate in decision making. However, if we are aware of it we may be able to avoid unnecessarily lengthy and detailed descriptions and discussions.

Finally, some patients may of course be *largely or totally incompetent* to make decisions because they are unconscious or confused, or perhaps just drowsy or muddled. Where their autonomy is severely compromised or absent because of the disease state they are completely at our mercy.

Given all these inequalities of power, no amount of patient 'empowerment', much in vogue at the present time, can eradicate the inevitable inequalities. No matter how much we try to enhance patient autonomy, we will always have relatively more than they have, given the special circumstances of palliative care.

Attempts have been made to reduce the inevitable inequalities of the relationship. For example, increasing importance is being placed on respecting patients' autonomy, sometimes even to the point of considering that this should be the overriding principle in health care (see Chapter 13, p. 278). In addition, patients are told that they can complain about the care they receive, and they know that they or their relatives can actually sue the carers if there is malpractice or negligence. However, does this really redress the balance of power in the palliative care situation, and could it ever do so given the circumstances? Patients are unlikely to complain about the carers on whom they are dependent, for fear that they may be discriminated against in the future. The patient is even less likely to sue the palliative care team because legal proceedings take so long that in the palliative care setting the patient is overwhelmingly likely to be dead before the case comes to court. It is unlikely that a distressed family would sue, partly because they are already stressed by dealing with their own grief, partly because a palliative care team is often surrounded by a halo effect due to obvious caring and good intentions, and partly because suing is likely to be difficult and traumatic when the key witness is dead. Finally, no amount of financial compensation can redress a wrong once the one who has suffered it is dead. Relatives are not likely to be motivated to sue the carers for wrongs committed against a deceased patient.

Thus the most striking feature of the carer–patient relationship is this inequality of power. However, despite this inequality in power, the patient and carer do share a strong motivation to achieve the patient's total good. In this respect they stand as it were 'side by side' and are drawn together.

Moreover, since a 'market economy' model for health care is now being developed in the United Kingdom's National Health Service, it has become more apparent that the carers rely on the patient's needs to justify their very existence. Thus the carers are dependent on the patient for their employment. In a sense this has always been true because the need of a society for doctors, nurses, and other health care workers is derived from the needs of the sick. Specialists in palliative care will continue to exist only if their particular expertise is seen to be needed and used by patients. In this way carers are dependent on patients for their professional role.

In summary we can say that the carer and patient stand in relative positions of great inequality of power. Whilst they share the same aim for the relationship, the carer has by far the greater ability to make this aim be realized. Ultimately, the carer has some of the 'goods' which the patient needs, but they must work together to ensure that such 'goods' as are chosen and provided are those most in accord with the patient's overall well-being or 'total good'.

Given the circumstances and features of the carer–patient relationship just described, are there any necessary conditions for the relationship to meet its stated aims? There are in fact two necessary moral conditions; the first is continued *commitment* to the patient's total good on behalf of the carer, and the second is *trust* in that commitment on behalf of the patient.

Are these conditions in fact sufficient for the success of the relationship? Unfortunately not, for many other factors are involved. For example, the carer must be competent, and the patient must be honest. It is important not to oversimplify this complex relationship by creating a model which is too simplistic. The two conditions mentioned, namely the carer's commitment to the patient's good and the patient's trust in it, are necessary precisely because of the unequal nature of the relationship.

The patient is forced to trust their doctor, nurse, or other health care worker. They have no choice but to trust the carer. Patients may choose their General Practitioner, but even then they cannot know exactly how competent or compassionate he or she is when that choice is made. In contrast, it is much more difficult for the patient to choose which hospital consultant, community nurse, or ward nurse will be involved, and frequently there is a very limited selection! It is always possible to seek a second opinion, but the patient's vulnerability to the second doctor is just as great as it was to the first. As a result of the patient's vulnerability, and the carer's possession and control of the needed knowledge, skills, and re-sources, the patient has no choice but to trust the professional. Once again, however much information about the illness and treatment the patient acquires, the carer will always have more. Trust in this relationship is ineradicable (Pellegrino and Thomasma 1988).

It follows that if patients are to be able to place this trust in their carers, then they must have some grounds for doing so. The best grounds for doing so are that the commitment to act for the patient's *total good* must be part of what it means to be a carer. As we have said, this ideal of beneficence must be more than a guiding principle, it must be intrinsic and therefore essential to being a carer. Unless this is understood by patients and carers alike, then there is no basis for the patient's trust, and it is clear that the requirement for trust in the relationship is ineradicable.

From this discussion the nature of the bond between the carer and patient begins to emerge. In a structural sense the purpose and substance of the bond is their shared aim, the patient's total good. Given the special characteristics of the patient and carer and their circumstances relative to each other, the achievement of that aim via the relationship is dependent on the carer's commitment to it and the patient's ability to trust in that commitment.

2.4 Models of the carer–patient relationship

It may be objected that some models for the carer–patient relationship claim to have diminished or abolished the need for trust on behalf of the patient, and commitment to our stated aim on behalf of the carer. We reject this claim and a brief study of these suggested models makes it clear that the trust and commitment described remain essential if the patient's good is to be served.

2.4.1   *Benevolent paternalism*

The traditional doctor–patient relationship was one of benevolent paternalism. In other words, doctors thought they should act in a loving and fatherly way towards their patients who were often ill-informed and uneducated. Inequalities of power related especially to knowledge were great and were acknowledged to be so. Doctors acted in the interests of the patient's medical good, and directed management towards what they considered as the patient's total good. The problem, of course, is that the patient cannot formulate ideas of his total good if not informed, and the doctor cannot have knowledge of that good unless he talks to the patient about it. Thus whilst this model probably furthered the patient's medical good, it did not necessarily provide care appropriate to the patient's total good. It has been rightly criticized because it tends to increase the likelihood of care being given which is contrary to the patient's overall well-being, which we have said is the ultimate aim of palliative care. In the traditional model the uninformed patient effectively had little autonomy in the first place, and the doctor did not feel it his duty to enhance this by providing information. Instead the doctor considered it most appropriate to reach his own con-clusions about the nature of the patient's medical and total good. Such an attitude has been described as paternalistic.

In general we have chosen to avoid using the words 'paternalism' and 'paternalistic' because of confusion in how they are used. But we can examine the traditional view without using such terms. Thus in our initial description of the traditional view of the doctor–patient relationship it can be seen that patients certainly placed ultimate trust in the doctor—indeed they were forced to by lack of infor-mation—but that trust was likely to be misplaced because the doctor was not then informed of the patient's perception of their own good. Whilst trust was present as a necessary condition of the relationship, commitment to the patient's own wishes was often lacking because the doctor practised in ignorance of them. This sometimes resulted in the almost exclusive pursuit of the patients' medical or biological good, often at the expense of their overall well-being or wholeness. Unfortunately, such a criticism of health care in general is still valid in some circumstances; life-sustaining and life-prolonging measures such as aggressive chemotherapy or resuscitation in dying patients are still sometimes used without regard for the patient's overall well-being.

More recently, alternative models for the carer–patient relationship have been proposed and their use is being increasingly encouraged in clinical practice, especially in palliative care. We could call these *autonomy-based models*. They vary according to whose autonomy is being emphasized; when it is that of the patient, the carer is seen simply as the agent enabling the patient's wishes to be fulfilled. When it is also that of the carer, then a contract model is proposed.

It is important to recognize that these models have emerged in an attempt to decrease the inequalities of power in the carer–patient relationship, and in support of each individual's right to self-determination. Whilst we feel that such an attempt is morally justified (because it emphasizes the unique value of each individual), it can never remove totally the imbalance of power. To the extent to which it is possible to achieve this, the autonomy-based models have been successful. However, we feel that the idea of equal power as a basis for the relationship is wrong and cannot work because equal power cannot be achieved for the reasons stated above. Nevertheless, we shall examine some autonomy-based models of the carer–patient relationship. In discussing these we shall recall the ambiguities in the concept of autonomy.

2.4.2   The customer–salesperson model

Recently in the UK there has been a political drive to run the National Health Service along the lines of a market economy, and in the USA health care funded by private insurance schemes already functions in this way. This has naturally led to the idea that the role of the patient equates with that of a 'customer', and that the role of the carer equates with that of a 'salesperson'. Without going into details of the moral nature of the customer–salesperson relationship, which is also undergoing change, it can be seen from commonly held attitudes such as 'the customer is always right' that the customer–salesperson relationship is not actually the same as the carer–patient relationship. We acknowledge that the salesperson does in fact have a duty of care to the customer. This normally entails explanation of the relative merits of items *if* requested—there is no duty to do so. It also entails warning the customer of potential dangers, and a duty to sell items which are fit for their purpose. However, ultimately the customer purchases what he or she wishes and at his or her own risk. Hence the common legal quote '*caveat emptor*' or 'the buyer beware'. The salesperson is not held morally responsible for the customer's purchase. This does not apply in palliative care where we hold carers morally (and legally) responsible for the care they deliver. The carer's task is to act for the patient's good, whereas the salesperson's aim is to sell goods.

For example, if the customer–salesperson model is applied in palliative care, then the doctor should describe all available treatments for the condition and their associated risks, benefits, and harms and the patient then simply chooses the treatment he or she wants. This would mean that a patient might choose to take a non-steroidal anti-inflammatory drug (NSAID) when there is a very high risk of gastrointestinal bleeding, or might choose surgery which is associated with a high mortality and morbidity, or might choose chemotherapy which has serious risks and harms and very little chance of benefit. According to the customer–salesperson model the doctor should provide whatever treatment the patient chooses, even if the doctor considers that in the particular clinical circumstances it is excessively risky or harmful or unlikely to be of benefit. Moreover, according to this model the patient bears responsibility for the choice, not the doctor, whose responsibility is confined to describing the benefits, risks, and harms of the treatments.

We do not feel that the customer–salesperson model, in which both parties are equally autonomous but the emphasis is on the customer's ends, is an appropriate model for the carer–patient relationship in palliative care. This is partly because many patients needing palliative care will at some time have severely compromised autonomy or none at all, and partly because the aims of the two relationships are actually different. The salesperson does not have a duty intrinsic to his or her role to act only for the customer's good, nor does the customer normally expect the salesperson to have such a commitment. Instead, the duty to sell the chosen item is intrinsic to the salesperson's role, and the ability to choose the desired item is intrinsic to the customer's role. This is not to denigrate morally the motivations and actions of salespersons or customers, but only to say that whilst they are appropriate to the aims of the customer–salesperson relationship, they are not appropriate for the carer–patient relationship in palliative care. A more detailed discussion on the problems of regarding respect for the patient's wishes as the overriding principle is given in Chapter 13, p. 278.

There is a real risk that carers, particularly doctors, will be insidiously persuaded by having to deliver health care through a market economy model that the customer–salesperson model is an appropriate one for their contact with patients. If this happens we believe that the good of the patient will no longer be served.

This risk is further increased by documents like the Patient's Charter (Department of Health 1995) which stress only the patient's right to choose care but not the carer's responsibility for delivering it. The fact that a patient chooses a certain treatment does not absolve the carer from the moral (or legal) responsibility for giving it.

2.4.3   *The contractual model*

This is a more logical approach in terms of the principle of respect for autonomy. It emphasizes and attempts to balance the autonomy of both the carer and the patient, mainly by laying down moral and legal rules of conduct. The moral rules tend to be implied or mutually understood but they do not take the form of a written contract. Nonetheless they are considered binding. The legal rules are written, and are familiar to all of us in the consent form.

Fortunately, the moral and legal rules concur and in this model they are very simple: no treatment can be given to a patient who is competent to make the decision if that patient refuses it, and no carer can be forced to give care or treatment which they strongly believe is not in the patient's best interests. In other words, no-one can force a patient to undergo treatment which the patient, if informed and competent, does not want, no matter what the consequences. No-one can force the carer to give treatment which he or she feels is contrary to the patient's good. Thus it is possible to stop both patient and carer from doing something, but not to make them do something. In other words, one can force an omission on the other party in the relationship, but one cannot force an action on the other party.

These rules exist to set limits to conduct where there is conflict between the autonomous choices of the carer and patient. However, setting limits is all these rules achieve; they do not help towards reaching a consensus decision by working together to establish the nature of the patient's total good. In a sense these rules are a minimalist policy to protect the autonomy of both parties. They actually do nothing to enhance the autonomy of either party.

Moreover, it could be argued that contracts are established between parties who feel they cannot necessarily trust each other. The contractual model is an attempt to decrease the need for trust on the patient's behalf. Yet we have said that trust is ineradicable in the carer–patient relationship. If the patient has to trust the carer, is there any need for a contract? What function does it serve? In fact it does protect the patient against the infliction of unwanted treatment, and it does protect the professional from having to act in a way which is contrary to his or her commitment to act for the patient's good. It is reasonable to conclude that the contractual model functions as a safeguard to both parties, but it is only a safeguard. It tells you how you must not act, but not how you should act.

The question as to who is responsible for most clinical management decisions is also unclear in this model. Fortunately, it is rare in the palliative care setting for a conflict to arise between patient and carer, such that either the carer absolutely refuses to give a certain treatment, and therefore takes full responsibility for the consequences of not giving it, or the patient absolutely refuses to undergo a recommended treatment, and therefore takes full responsibility for the consequences of not having it. The contractual model stipulates only who has moral responsibility in these two uncommon circumstances. It leaves us wondering who has moral responsibility for the consequences of the majority of clinical decisions which are actually made following mutual discussion.

It has another serious shortcoming, especially in palliative care—it is applicable only to autonomous patients (and perhaps to non-autonomous ones who have left advance directives—a rare document at the time of writing). Terminally ill patients, as we have said, often have compromised autonomy because of anxiety, fear, extreme weakness, and depression. All of these plus exhaustion can make them more easily coerced by others. Dying patients may undergo a period of mild to moderate confusion or drowsiness prior to unconsciousness and death. Many of our patients will therefore have severely compromised or no autonomy for some of the time they are in our care, and the contractual model is not applicable at these times.

In conclusion, whilst the contractual model is a help in a minimalist way, it is inadequate alone as a model of conduct for the patient–carer relationship in palliative care.

2.4.4 The partnership model

We have said that the aim of the relationship is the patient's total good, which encompasses the intrinsic and the extrinsic aims of palliative care. The patient knows his or her own life plans, values and priorities, whilst the carer knows how best to achieve what we have called the patient's medical good in a biological sense. The patient's total good can be served only by sharing of knowledge between the patient and carer because that total good is achieved only by combination of the medical good with the patient's goals and values. Therefore, the only appropriate relationship between them is one of partnership, where both work together towards their mutual goal.

In the partnership model the aim is achieved by working together. Since the autonomy of both patient and carer is involved, and this entails each determining and governing their own responses to the other, both share responsibility for decisions which are reached. To the extent that each exercises his or her autonomy, they are each responsible for the decision. This is in contrast to the consumerist approach embodied in the customer–salesperson model in which the carer can abdicate responsibility for the decision and therefore for the outcome. We feel that such an approach encourages the carer to abdicate from the entire responsibility for the decision by passing it to the patient, and whilst this may appear attractive (particularly with the rising possibility of litigation), we consider that it amounts to moral abandonment by the professional (Pellegrino and Thomasma 1988).

The idea of working together with patients in planning care has always been part of the philosophy of palliative care, but the partnership model for the carer–patient relationship shares some of the shortcomings of the customer–salesperson and contractual models in that it assumes that the patient is largely autonomous, and at times in palliative care this is definitely not the case. If an attitude of respect for the patient's own life plans and direction of management towards the patient's total good are appropriate for the autonomous patient, what attitude is appropriate for the non-autonomous patient? In the absence of an advance statement by the patient, we cannot know of the patient's own ends, values, or chosen life plans.

2.4.5   *The trustee model*

To cover the case where the patient is deteriorating and is increasingly incapable of expressing a view on her own good, we require to introduce another model. The model of the trustee fits many aspects of this situation. A trustee is someone who acts in the best interests of another when the other cannot act for herself, perhaps because of immaturity or senility or death. The trustee will always take into account whatever is known of the wishes of the party in question, and will at all times act for her best interests. Carrying over the model into palliative care we use our professional knowledge base to plan and deliver care in accordance with the patient's medical good, but this management plan is then modified by any knowledge we may be able to gain about the patient's view of his or her total good. As far as possible care should still be directed towards whatever we know of the patient's perception of overall well-being. As we become less able to reach decisions with the patient because her autonomy is declining and it becomes increasingly difficult to ascertain what her wishes might be, so we must act progressively more in accordance with the attitudes of compassion and beneficence, and direct care towards her medical good.

It can be seen that the concept of an attitude is particularly useful in palliative care, whose philosophy we have said is based on a whole person perspective of the patient. It seems right therefore that the morality of the carer should also be viewed from a whole person perspective which embraces our beliefs, our emotions, and our behaviour. Therefore, the use of attitudes as a way of describing morality in palliative care is both appropriate and helpful.

We have looked at various models of the carer–patient relationship. Each has some truth but no one model can express the full nature of the relationship, because patients and their medical conditions vary so much. Nevertheless, the moral principles and virtues we discussed in Chapter 1 were seen to underlie and structure the relationship.

2.5 Consent

These models of the patient–carer relationship have a logical bearing on appropriate ways of seeking consent to treatment. There are three senses of the term 'consent' which should be considered in the context of health care.

2.5.1 Consent as in accepting

The weakest sense of consent is 'agreeing to' or 'accepting'. If we take an analogy from consent in political philosophy: then a ruler like Elizabeth I of England ruled by consent in that she was popular and the populace accepted or agreed with her policies of beating up the Spanish, etc. But her *right* to act in this way did not depend on their agreement; if they had not agreed, then it would not have mattered. This is the weakest sense of consent. In medicine it might be illustrated in contexts in which the doctor says 'I am proposing to do X and Y' or 'I have just done X and Y. Is that OK?', and the patient weakly says 'Yes, thank you doctor'. This strand of the consent doctrine is compatible with the main tradition in that it does not confer rights on the patient. This sense of consent is related to the model of benevolent paternalism.

2.5.2 Consent as in authorizing

A strong sense of consent is 'authorizing'. A might authorize B to do X, Y on his behalf. In this case B's *right* to do X, Y derives from A, and the main responsibility for the doing of X and Y rests with A. For example, I might instruct or authorize my agent to bid for me at an auction, or the patient might authorize the doctor to provide a certain treatment. This is too strong a sense of consent to be assimilated into even a modified main tradition in medical ethics. It has the serious disadvantage in medicine of undermining professional autonomy: the doctor may feel that what the patient authorizes is futile, and in any case it is up to the doctor to make the treatment decisions (although, as we shall see, the patient can legitimately refuse treatment). It should be noted that the use of the term 'directive' as in 'advance directive' may encourage patients to see themselves as authorizing their doctor to act as their agent. But the term 'directive' means what it says only if the patient is refusing treatment. The patient may suggest or permit treatment but cannot authorize it.

Contrary to our US colleagues there is good reason for maintaining the asymmetry whereby the patient may legitimately refuse a treatment or authorize a refusal, but cannot authorize, as distinct from agree to, the positive giving of a treatment. The explanation is that the doctor is the expert on the patient's *medical* good—hence only the doctor can authorize treatment—but the patient is the expert on his or her own *total* good. In the light of this knowledge of an overall or total good, the patient is entitled to *refuse* treatment which might well be in his or her narrower medical good. This sense of consent as authorizing is related to the customer–salesperson model.

2.5.3 Consent as shared decision making

Shared decision making has two elements:

(i) Patient preferences and values are discussed with the doctor in the light of the doctor's treatment proposals or they could be mentioned in advance in a document. This type of discussion is necessary but not sufficient for what we are calling joint or shared decision making.

(ii) The second necessary condition is that this discussion results in the activating of a socially or often a legally sanctioned procedure. We can call this procedure the giving or the refusing of *permission*. These two conditions are together necessary and sufficient for this sense of consent. We should like to note some points about it.

   (a) Permission is given by both patient and doctor. Each may permit treatment or not.

   (b) Permission is a *normative* term. It is not like 'agreeing' or 'accepting' which are non-normative—I can accept a drink or agree to go to the cinema without any question of *rights*. But to give permission is to confer a right. Thus the patient gives or refuses the doctor a right to intervene, and the doctor gives the patient the right to have or not to have the treatment in question.

(c) The norms in question must be socially and in the end legally sanctioned or legitimized by public policy. In other words, the parties must know and agree about procedures, and *society* more generally must know and agree.

Shared decision making seems the most satisfactory model for consent in the clinical situation. This sense of consent has elements of the contractual model and the partnership model. There are, however, three difficulties with this solution.

The first will arise if the patient or relatives persist in requesting a certain treatment which the doctor thinks is not appropriate. There cannot in this situation be shared decision making. This creates a challenge to the doctor's ability to communicate with the patient and relatives. The vast majority of patients will in the end accept the doctor's advice. In the rare situation in which the doctor's advice is not accepted then the doctor must hold firmly to his professional judgement, and in this as we have seen the doctor will be supported, at least in the UK, in the courts. In this case the doctor is taking sole responsibility for the decision not to carry out the treatment.

The second difficulty concerns a possible shift from the idea that a patient has a right to give informed consent to the idea that the patient has a duty to do so. In the latter case the giving of informed consent becomes a precondition of receiving any treatment. We can understand why this view may gain ground—it protects the doctor from the threats of litigation and criticism—but we think it is undesirable in most spheres of medicine and in particular it is undesirable in palliative care. The reason it is undesirable in palliative care is that it would force patients to be fully informed about the effects of treatment on the course of the illness, which would entail a discussion about possible future symptoms and about ways of dying. Not all patients would want to be forced to confront these realities, but they are surely entitled to receive treatment. Hence there is still some room, at least in palliative care, for the weak sense of consent as simply accepting the treatment advised. This solution to the issue of consent is related to the model of benevolent paternalism.

The third difficulty arises with respect to those patients who are not capable of making their own decisions. Many patients in the context of palliative care will at some time be incapable of giving informed consent by reason of confusion, unconsciousness, etc. Most will not have indicated in advance their preferences regarding treatment in the circumstances which actually arise. Their care then most appropriately falls under the trustee model described in Section 2.4.5 above.

2.6 Conclusions

1. The nature of the carer–patient relationship is determined by its aims; the intrinsic aim is the relief of suffering due to physical or mental illness, and extrinsic aims are relief of psychological, social, and spiritual distress.

2. A major feature of the relationship is inequality of power; the carer has the knowledge, skills, and resources which the patient needs. Therefore, trust on behalf of the patient is an ineradicable feature of the relationship.

3. Commitment to the patient's well-being or wholeness (termed 'total good') is called an attitude of beneficence and is intrinsic to the role of carer. On the basis of professional knowledge the carer proposes management in accordance with the patient's biological or medical good.

4. Various models of the relationship were examined and were found to be in different ways satisfactory, or unsatisfactory, depending on the circumstances and condition of the patient.

5. Three senses of the concept of consent were examined, and that of shared decision making where both parties give permission was found to be the most satisfactory, but is still not appropriate for all circumstances.

3

The relative–professional relationship

If a man's character is to be abused, say what you will, there's nobody like a relative to do the business.
W. M. Thackeray, *Vanity Fair*, Ch. 19

Where there is officialdom every human relationship suffers.
E. M. Forster, *Passage to India*, Ch. 24

In this chapter consideration is given to the nature and appropriate conduct of the relationship between professional carers and the patient's family or other close friends, referred to in general terms as 'relatives'. This relationship is referred to as the relative–professional relationship, in order to avoid confusion surrounding the word 'carer' which we used to denote a professional carer in Chapter 2, but which is sometimes used to denote a friend or family member who is looking after the patient.

We have said that the intrinsic aim of palliative care is the patient's 'medical good', which comprises the amelioration of the disease process, the prolongation of life, and the relief of suffering. This intrinsic aim is achieved through the patient–professional carer relationship and by means of the professional knowledge-base and skills of medicine, nursing, social work, and allied health professions. In contrast, we have said that the promotion of the patient's psychological good is an extrinsic aim of palliative care. In Chapter 1 we stated that to include the care of relatives within the intrinsic aim of palliative care is inappropriate for two reasons. Firstly, it is unrealistic because the resources required for patient care are already stretched. Secondly, unresolvable conflicts of interest between the needs of the patients and those of the relatives are inevitable if the care of relatives is seen as part of the intrinsic aim of palliative care. However, we did suggest that supporting relatives by means of humane practical wisdom is a reasonable extrinsic aim of palliative care.

Yet in palliative care it is sometimes said that 'the unit of care is the family', thus making the 'care' of relatives part of the professionals' aim and suggesting that professionals have obligations towards the relatives. However, if this is the case, unresolvable conflicts of interest must arise between patients and their relatives and then a choice must be made between meeting the patient's wants and needs and those of the relatives. Analysis of the moral nature of the relationship between professionals and relatives is necessary in order to determine whether there are obligations which professionals have towards relatives, and to determine how we should act when conflicts of interest arise between patients and relatives. As with the patient–professional carer relationship, the nature of the role link between relatives and professionals will be considered. Suggestions can then be made about appropriate attitudes—ways of thinking and behaving—which professionals should have towards relatives.

By analysing the relative–professional relationship we do not wish to denigrate in any way the bonds of love and kinship which link patients and their friends and family, and we acknowledge the moral importance of these bonds. But the existence of close bonds between patient and relative does not mean that professionals should extend to the patient's family the special role relationship which exists between patient and health care professional.

There are three aspects of the role relationship between health care professionals and relatives. Firstly, they may both act as carers for the patient and so share this responsibility. Secondly, they may both have a part to play in decision making regarding aspects of care and treatment. Thirdly, since relatives are in intimate relationships with patients, patients and relatives are bound to affect each other in psychological and physical ways. Does it follow from this that the professional has duties to the relatives for the sake of the patient? Lastly, we must ask whether any of these three aspects of the role relationship establishes direct duties or obligations towards relatives.

3.1   The relatives as co-carers

The family and close friends of patients are usually involved in aspects of the patient's physical care and psychological support during the illness. Together with professionals they are carers of the patient. This role link is then one of partnership. Professionals have the knowledge and skills, whilst relatives have the time, motivation, and with guidance the practical ability to care for the patient.

This partnership role usually works well and gives rise to few moral problems because it is generally accepted both that relatives can provide some physical care and advice, and that their wishes should not prevail if physical harm to the patient is likely to result. Nevertheless, there are contexts when conflicts of interest can occur.

3.1.1 *Relatives and patients causing each other harm*

Occasionally, circumstances arise when relatives are caring for patients such that they may cause each other harm, usually because of a conflict of interest between them. Only very rarely is the harm intentional. Health care professionals find themselves in the position of trying to minimize harm to either party. The following examples illustrate familiar problems.

Firstly, relatives who are caring for the patient at home occasionally wish to prevent doctors and nurses from having access to the patient. This may happen because the relatives are unable to accept the severity of the illness and want to prevent the involvement of a palliative care team because allowing it forces them to acknowledge the seriousness of the illness.

Secondly, they may resent the entry of strangers into their home, and so wish to prevent professionals from coming in to treat the patient.

Thirdly, families may wish to prevent the patient from learning the nature of the illness and may refuse to permit specialist palliative care teams into the house because they fear that the presence of such a team will inform the patient about the true nature of the illness. In these situations explanation to and negotiation with the relatives nearly always results in their permitting access to the patient. However, if these measures fail it is generally accepted that relatives should not be able to deny the patient access to essential health care services, and so legal measures exist to remove the patient to a 'place of safety', such as a hospital, in order to provide essential care. However, it must be acknowledged that the professionals require courage and energy to use whatever legal measures are at their disposal to ensure that in these rare situations the patient receives essential care. They should be committed to the view that access to such care should not be blocked by the family.

Fourthly, it occasionally happens that relatives undertaking physical care of the patient sometimes want to undertake procedures harmful to the patient. For example, it is not uncommon for relatives to wish to try to give oral food or fluids when patients are exceedingly weak or semi-conscious and their swallowing reflex is impaired. Aspiration of the food or fluids into the lungs is then likely and is very hazardous and possibly unpleasant for the patient. The relatives' desire to provide nutrition and hydration is usually based on the belief that it will either enhance the patient's comfort or prolong life. It is generally accepted that relatives must be dissuaded from actions such as this which are very likely to cause physical harm to the patient.

It should be clear from these four situations that when misguided relatives wish to pursue a course of action which is likely to result in physical harm to the patient, such harm must be prevented, even if this means frustrating the wishes and goals of the relatives. Whilst professionals know what they ought to do in this situation, we must repeat that facing up to the conflict is difficult and sometimes unpleasant, and courage combined with willingness to spend time speaking firmly but tactfully to the relatives is required. It is much easier not to intervene and risk harm to the patient.

There can also be situations where granting the wishes of patients would result in a significant risk of serious physical harm to the relatives. For example, patients frequently prefer to be lifted by one or two people rather than by a hoist, but the risks to relatives of lifting are well known. In this situation health care professionals should insist to the patient that such lifting is hazardous to the relatives and that a hoist should be used. Relatives may also be exposed to risks of serious harm if HIV positive patients do not want their HIV status to be disclosed and so request professionals to keep this information confidential. Fortunately, this occurs only very rarely as most patients appreciate the justice of informing their relatives in order that the latter should not be exposed to the risk of infection. Even if the patient declines to permit disclosure, there are grounds for the health care professional to breach confidentiality because it is necessary to do so in order to prevent a significant risk of serious harm to the relatives. In the absence of a cure for AIDS, infection with the HIV virus must certainly be considered a serious harm.

In the above examples it is clear that we do not consider it acceptable for the professionals to comply with the relatives' wishes if physical harm to the patient is likely to ensue. Nor do we consider that we should comply with the patient's wishes if physical harm to the relatives is likely to ensue.

3.1.2   Conflicts regarding place of care

Perhaps the most common conflict of interest between relatives and patients which might damage the interests of either arises concerning the issue of whether relatives feel willing and able to care for the patient at home. This causes conflicts of interest regarding the place of care for the patient. Relatives are of course free to decide how much care they feel able to give the patient although such decisions are often morally difficult for them. They feel under an obligation to offer care because of the bonds of kinship and also because the patient is frequently sharing the same accommodation and has immediately apparent needs which at times only the relative is on hand to meet. Many relatives become exhausted emotionally and physically, and yet find it difficult to be honest about their increasing reluctance to shoulder what has become a heavy burden of care. At other times, and especially where relationships have been less than loving, relatives do not want to undertake physical care for the patient, or are afraid of the consequences of having the very sick and possibly dying patient at home. Relatives in these situations often need the support of professionals to be honest with the patient about their feelings.

However, professionals cannot remove the responsibility for these difficult decisions from relatives, for no-one can relieve another of the moral ties of kinship. Relatives sometimes ask professionals to mislead patients by inventing a medical reason for admission to hospital, when in fact the reason for such a move is because the relatives feel unable and/or unwilling to continue caring for the patient, even with assistance from outside agencies. In this situation it is tempting for professionals to comply, yet it is morally preferable to insist that the relatives are honest about their feelings, and if appropriate to explain to the patient that the relatives' exhaustion is real and understandable. It is also usually possible to describe honestly any medical advantages of a move to hospital, specialist palliative care unit, or other residential care.

It is clear that professionals do not have an obligation to mislead patients in order to avoid difficult decisions and situations for relatives. Indeed, it can be said that professionals have an obligation not to mislead either party, but especially the patient, because it is the patient's responsibility to make a decision about a move into residential care and to make such decisions competent patients need accurate information.

It is easy for professionals to be seen to 'take sides' in this particular conflict of interests, either on behalf of the patient or the relatives. When patients are weak and exhausted it is sometimes necessary to encourage them to assert their point of view, and perhaps to explain the patient's position to relatives. But ultimately, conflicts of this nature need to be resolved by the patients and relatives together, since each bears responsibility for their decisions. Professional carers have an obligation to give information and advice about matters related to the illness, within the constraints of confidentiality, but they are under no obligation to impose a solution on the parties involved in this common situation. Instead, relatives and patient need to come to an agreement together. If agreement cannot be reached, then each side has a fall-back position; competent patients can refuse to move into residential care from their homes, and relatives can refuse to continue to provide care. Fortunately, in a climate of open discussion with willingness to review the decision it is very rare for an amicable solution not to be found.

The moral problem regarding place of care is obviously different if the patient is incompetent and unable to state his or her wishes. Whilst a competent patient can refuse admission to hospital (unless legally forced to do so under the provisions of the Mental Health Act), an incompetent patient is not able to refuse to get into an ambulance, although the patient may have previously expressed wishes with regard to place of care. Under UK law it is clear that the responsibility of health care professionals is to act in the patient's (not the relative's) best interests, and the law in this case effectively gives professionals the role of guardians of the patient's best interests. Making judgements about the patient's best interests is obviously difficult and complex in that many factors need to be taken into account. Morally relevant factors include whether the patient's care and treatment needs can be adequately met at home by the relatives and/or professional care agencies, and also the patient's previously stated wishes. This reflects the description of best interests as being derived from the patient's medical good and ascertainable wishes. The following examples help to illustrate this point.

An elderly frail and terminally ill lady was being looked after by her daughter in her daughter's home. The palliative care team were asked by the GP to visit with a view to ongoing contact, and at the first visit it became clear that her daughter was tired and requested respite admission. The patient agreed to this on the condition that she would return to her daughter's home again and would die there, as was her wish. Her daughter did not intimate that there was any problem with this and agreed that she would look after her mother again after respite care, which was then arranged a few days ahead. The patient's condition deteriorated suddenly over the intervening weekend with signs of bronchopneumonia and the on-call GP telephoned to ask for admission of the patient to the palliative care unit as her daughter had said she could not bear the thought of the patient's death in her house, and would feel afterwards that she could not bear to live there. The patient was moribund and not distressed or in pain and it was clearly not in her medical interests to be moved at that stage. Moreover, her previously expressed wish had been to be in her daughter's home—a wish expressed when she was under the impression that her daughter was willing to look after her. The patient was transferred to the palliative care unit and fortunately survived the journey, although she died within 6 hours, without distress. According to this patient's best interests she should not have been moved. It may be argued that her expressed wish to remain in the home should be disregarded as she was not aware that her daughter did not want to look after her. On the other hand, we are not in a position to know what she would have wanted if she had known this, especially as she had been unwilling to contemplate the idea of not returning after respite care to die at home. It is almost impossible to surmise what her wishes might have been in the circumstances which actually arose and which there was no evidence to suggest she had foreseen. Consequently, we would argue that her medical good only can be known, and this was not served by transfer to the palliative care unit. The only possible justification for her transfer is that she was in her daughter's home, and that her daughter may have had a right to insist she no longer remained there—although this does seem a very weak justification. The true explanation of her transfer, and many similar transfers, is that it is easier to transfer the incompetent patient who cannot complain than to confront the relative's problems and refuse to move the patient. The issue of any possible obligation to 'avoid harm to' the relative or to 'respect her autonomy' in this situation is addressed later.

Similar considerations arise in making a best interests judgement regarding discharge of an incompetent patient from hospital. Once again, it can be very difficult or impossible to surmise what the patient's wishes would have been in the circumstances which have actually arisen. The circumstances which actually arise are rarely those which the patient envisaged and commented upon, and it can be difficult to extrapolate accurately from the patient's stated wishes about one situation to a view on the patient's probable wishes in another situation. When a reasonably accurate judgement cannot be made about the patient's wishes in the actual circumstances, it seems to us that the patient's medical good should be served since it is the only aspect of best interests which can be known.

3.2   The relatives as decision makers

We stated earlier that the extent to which relatives should be involved in making decisions on behalf of patients is contentious. This issue can be discussed in terms of three situations: decision making by parents on behalf of young children, decision making by relatives on behalf of incompetent adult patients, and decision making by relatives on behalf of competent patients. It is helpful to consider in each situation the grounds for relatives having decision-making responsibility, and to compare those grounds when justifying our conclusions.

At the start it is helpful to remind ourselves that logically a relative ought not to have greater authority in health care decisions than a competent patient has. The competent patient can consent to or refuse any treatment offered, but cannot demand a treatment which the health care team consider is clinically inappropriate or which cannot be resourced. Thus the maximum decision-making power a relative could hold would be to consent to or refuse a treatment on behalf of the patient, but the relative could not demand a treatment which the health care team consider clinically inappropriate or which could not be resourced. The most power a relative could hold would be that which a patient holds.

3.2.1   *Parental decision making on behalf of young children*

It is widely agreed that parents have a right to make health care decisions on behalf of young children and infants. It is important to analyse the grounds of such a right, in order to ascertain its scope.

For example, it is helpful to consider if and when that parental right should be overridden by a public body such as a court.

Infants and young children are not competent to make health care decisions for themselves, and so there must be a proxy or surrogate decision maker. It is readily assumed that the parents should adopt this role, but why?

One obvious ground, and that most often cited, is that parents will decide according to their child's best interests. This is based on two assumptions; firstly, that because of their constant and close relationship parents know their child's best interests, and secondly, that because of the strong and unselfish love which parents typically have for their children they will actually decide in the child's best interests. These assumptions and the conclusion based upon them are open to dispute.

Firstly, parents will never have as much knowledge of the medical situation as the paediatricians and other members of the health care team, and in the case of sick children the medical interests are likely to be the best interests. It is therefore contestable that parents always have a better understanding of their child's best interests than others who have extensive experience of the illness and similar clinical circumstances.

Secondly, parents have to make decisions based on the welfare of the whole family unit. They may have several children, and the best interests of the sick child may have to be set aside in favour of the other children or some other family good. Parents also have duties in addition to those to their children. For example, they have duties to each other, to their own parents, employers, and so forth. Their decisions are influenced by their duties to the whole family group. Thus, whereas a child's best interests may often be identified with those of the family unit, this is not always the case. The optimum treatment and care for the sick child may have to be subordinated to the good or responsibilities of other family members. For example, occasionally parents may decline life-prolonging treatment for a disabled child because of the impact of that child's care needs on the whole family. Again, sometimes religious beliefs can lead parents to decline treatment which most people would consider to be in the child's best interests.

Thirdly, parents may sometimes request life-prolonging treatment which in their child's case is excessively burdensome because they cannot bear the thought of losing their child. They may request or demand treatment which is very unpleasant and where the chances of improved survival are remote. They may want all possible treatments tried which might prolong life because they are tormented by feelings of guilt if they fail to pursue all such measures.

Thus it is contestable that the ground for a parental right of decision making is that parents are the people most likely to make the decision which accords with the child's best interests; whilst it is in general the case that parents will decide in the child's best interests, it is not always so.

Another way of seeing a parental right to decide on behalf of children might be a sort of ownership or property right. Yet this is intuitively unattractive, for the phrase 'this is my child' does not indicate an ownership relationship. Contemporary morality is totally opposed to the notion that any human being actually has ownership or property rights over another.

Since we cannot ground the parental right either in the child's best interests criterion or in an ownership criterion, we must look elsewhere for the grounds of the parental right. It is more plausibly seen in the activity of parenting.

Parenting itself is seen to have a special value in society, because of the opportunity it gives to express an unselfish love, and to cherish and nurture the child from infancy to maturity, passing on traditions and values. People very much want to become parents, demonstrating that it is an activity which is greatly valued in itself, and not just because it is socially necessary as a way of rearing the children who will continue the human race. The parent–child relationship is undoubtedly an intimate relationship, and one in which parents usually show devotion to the child's welfare, even at the expense of their own. The language of rights and duties between parent and child seems inappropriate and inadequate in the context of such a relationship. But since it is commonly used, it is reasonable to conclude that the right of parents to make health care decisions on behalf of their children is grounded in and justified by the need to preserve the intimate relationship that is parenthood. It is a right against interference by other bodies, and that right is seen as justified by the need to protect and promote the valuable role of parenting in society. It is to do with preserving and stressing the ideal of this intimate relationship within the family.

However, this right to freedom from external intervention is not and never could be absolute. Doctors can and should decline to give treatments which are inappropriate because they entail harms which are excessive in comparison with the possible benefits, or treatments which will consume so many resources that other patients will be deprived of more beneficial treatments as a result. In fact, children are often given treatments which have very little chance of success for the justifiable reason that if they are effective and a cure is achieved the gain may be many years of life. On the other hand, such treatments may be given because of the emotive content of 'life-saving' treatment for children, especially as expressed in the media, and because it is so difficult for doctors to deny a treatment to parents who are demanding it for their child. These latter reasons are not moral justifications, but they are explanations regarding the use of treatments which entail major harms and very little likelihood of significant benefit, and which are regarded as medically inappropriate.

On the other hand, when parents refuse a life-saving treatment, such as a blood transfusion for a child of parents who are Jehovah's Witnesses, application to the court may be made by health care professionals and the court may override parental refusal of treatment. This procedure exists in acknowledgement of the fact that parents may not always decide in the best interests of their child, and so mechanisms are necessary to override parental refusal of life-saving treatment in cases where the parental view is widely regarded as unreasonable. However, in the interests of preserving the intimate relationship of parenthood, intervention by the courts is made only when parental refusal of treatment is clearly unreasonable and the cost is likely to be the life of the child.

Thus, in general, parents are rightly granted decision-making authority for their young children. Therefore, when the health care team offer treatment for their child, parents may accept or decline it. In this respect the parent–professional relationship bears a close resemblance to the patient–professional carer relationship described in Chapter 2.

3.2.2 Relatives' decision making on behalf of incompetent adults

Individual opinions and the policies of different countries vary on the question of whether relatives should have legal decision-making responsibilities, rights, or duties for incompetent adults. For example, in the United Kingdom no adult can legally consent to or refuse treatment on behalf of another adult (unless appointed as a proxy) and so health care professionals make decisions based on a best interests judgement, which is informed by what can be known of the patient's previously expressed wishes. In other countries relatives are given decision-making powers in that they can consent to or refuse treatment on behalf of incompetent adults. As previously stated, relatives do not and should not have power to demand inappropriate treatment for patients.

It might be suggested that relatives should have decision-making powers because they are the people most likely to decide in accordance with the patient's best interests. This claim rests on the same assumptions as were relevant to the parents of young children; firstly, that relatives are most likely to know the patient's best interests because of familiarity with the patient's personality, wishes, and values, and secondly, that relatives will actually decide in the patient's best interests. Both these assumptions are contestable.

Health care professionals may be better placed than relatives to make judgements about the patient's medical good. This is because they will always have more information about the clinical circumstances of the illness. They will always have a better understanding, based on theory and experience, of the benefits and harms of treatments and of the likely course of the illness with and without certain treatments. Whilst relatives will inevitably know more about the patient's wishes and values, this knowledge forms only part of a best interests judgement. The remainder relates to medical good and is a matter of clinical knowledge which the health care team will always possess to a greater extent than the relatives. Thus the patient's medical good, which is always a major factor in a best interests judgement, is better known by the health care team than the relatives. Therefore, it cannot be assumed that relatives are better placed to make a judgement of the patient's best interests than the health care team.

Moreover, it is inevitable that relatives have many interests of their own, and these may conflict with the patient's best interests. Whilst parental love is typically unselfish and even self-denying, the relationships between spouses or other relatives are much more varied in nature. Most parents will tend to place their child's interests on a par with or above their own, but this is not true to the same extent of adult–adult relationships. Relatives may have major financial interests at stake, especially as the care of dependent patients consumes more and more of the patient's and family's resources. Moreover, the care of a sick adult relative is more likely to be seen as burdensome than the care of one's sick child, partly because it is physically often more difficult, and partly because we expect and accept the duty to care for and nurture our children but we do not have the same attitude towards care for our sick adult relatives. Thus it is by no means clear that relatives will be sufficiently unselfish to choose in the patient's best interests. To expect this would be to expect an almost heroic degree of effacement of personal interests.

Since it cannot be assumed that relatives will make those decisions most in accordance with the patient's best interests, this assumption cannot serve as justification for granting them decision-making powers.

It is true that someone must make decisions on behalf of incompetent patients, and it is contestable that the health care team is more likely to make decisions in accordance with the patients best interests. However, on balance it is considered in some communities, such as the United Kingdom, that health care professionals are more likely to make such decisions than relatives. On the other hand, as health care resources become further stretched, and professionals become increasingly responsible for rationing treatment and care, this assumption should be questioned. This issue is discussed further in Chapter 12 on resource allocation.

The suggestion that an idea of ownership or property right should serve as a justification for decision-making powers for relatives of adult patients is intuitively unattractive. The idea of ownership of one adult by another is repugnant in modern society.

It might be argued, as in the case of infants and young children, that relatives should have a right and possibly a duty to make health care decisions for incompetent adult patients in order to protect and promote the value and privacy of intimate relationships. Whilst this could be argued for spouses and other first-degree relatives, it is less convincing in the case of more distant relatives who have less contact and intimacy with the patient. Moreover, there may be disadvantages to relatives if they were given decision-making authority for patients as a matter of public policy. For example, if they were considered to have a right to make decisions for incompetent patients, they would logically also have to take their share of responsibility for those decisions. Furthermore, the right to make such decisions might come to be seen as a duty. Then many relatives might find the duty and responsibility for making such decisions very burdensome. They might suffer feelings of guilt whatever they decided, especially with regard to decisions regarding life-prolonging or life-sustaining treatment, or where palliative treatments offered to alleviate suffering might foreseeably shorten life. Thus a public policy which gave decision-making powers to relatives would force relatives to take significant responsibility for medically complex and morally difficult decisions. Many relatives would be reluctant to undertake this task, and would prefer that this responsibility be passed on to the health care team, whilst their role in informing the team of the patient's wishes and values is maintained. Thus in the case of decision making for incompetent adults the disadvantages to the relatives of giving them decision-making authority may outweigh the social benefit of acknowledging and protecting the privacy of intimate relationships.

On the other hand, it may be argued that there are practical grounds for passing decision-making responsibility to relatives when the adult patient is incompetent. For example, it has been suggested that litigation by relatives may be reduced if they, rather than the health care team, bear decision-making responsibility for incompetent adult patients. For whenever health care professionals make a decision based on the patient's best interests, which always contains some value judgements open to varying opinion, there exists the possibility that relatives may disagree with the judgement and choose to sue the health care team. If this occurs it is overwhelmingly likely that the patient will be either dead or incapable of acting as a witness in the proceedings.

The perceived threat of the expense and trauma of such litigation can coerce health care professionals into acting against the patients interests but according to the relatives' wishes. Moreover, in the UK the costs of litigation are born by the National Health Service, thus directly reducing the funds available for patient care. The overall result is that health care professionals are very much tempted to accede to the relatives' wishes, even if they believe that to do so may harm the patient, in order to minimize the possibility of unpleasant and costly litigation.

It is plausible that making the relatives responsible for decisions regarding incompetent adults would significantly reduce both the threat of litigation and its costs. Such a solution might also be attractive to health care professionals because it would allow them to escape the difficult task of making decisions for incompetent patients, and then taking responsibility for those decisions. Despite these suggested advantages, in the UK relatives do not have legal powers to consent to or refuse treatment on behalf of incompetent adult patients. This public policy exists because currently it is considered that the good of incompetent patients is best served if decisions regarding their care are made by the health care team, and not by their relatives. The law effectively backs up the judgement of health care professionals, in order that they should have the courage to make those treatment decisions which they consider most accord with the patient's best interests, even if in some cases the relatives' wishes are not granted.

We conclude from this discussion that the suggested grounds for giving decision-making powers to the relatives of incompetent patients fail to justify such a policy. On balance, the disadvantages for both patients and relatives of giving decision-making authority and responsibility to relatives seem to us to outweigh the advantages. However, in other countries with significant cultural differences and ways of resourcing treatment and care the balance may in fact fall in favour of granting decision-making responsibility to the relatives.

3.2.3 Relatives' decision making on behalf of competent adults

It is generally agreed in Western cultures that competent patients should make their own decisions regarding treatment. In so doing they will usually choose to discuss relevant issues with chosen family members, and may well take the interests of the family into account. However, it is also generally agreed that patients should not be coerced by relatives when making decisions.

Given the general level of agreement about this issue it is somewhat surprising that health care professionals will still sometimes withhold essential information from patients who want it—for example, knowledge of the diagnosis—at the request of relatives. The explanation for this practice is probably that it is simply easier to accede to the wishes of highly assertive relatives than to face confrontation. Whilst this is an explanation, it is not adequate as a justification of this practice. In many countries the law upholds the right of patients to information about their illnesses, yet this information is still sometimes withheld from patients because health care professionals lack the courage and energy to override the relatives' wishes. Whatever the relationship between relatives and professionals should be, it definitely should not be one of conspiracy to conceal information about the illness and treatments from a patient who wants or needs it.

Advance statements are sometimes made by competent patients to indicate their wishes with regard to treatment when they are incompetent. They very often contain advance refusals of certain treatments, or a general statement that in certain circumstances they would not want life-prolonging or life-sustaining treatment. Relatives may wish to override an advance refusal of treatment. Yet we would wish to argue that they should not be able to override a refusal which is valid, i.e. was competently made, and which is applicable, i.e. was intended to apply to the circumstances which have actually arisen. It is possible that advance refusals which are valid and applicable may become legally binding in the UK, in order to prevent their being overridden either by relatives or health care professionals. Whilst there are disadvantages in making advance refusals legally binding, such as the practical problems of establishing validity and applicability and the inability to ascertain whether the patient might have changed his or her mind, legal force may be necessary to prevent health care professionals and relatives from overriding those refusals. The overriding of such refusals by health care professionals and relatives constitutes the overriding of the wishes of the now non-autonomous patient by the autonomous professionals and relatives. One important function of the law is to uphold the rights and interests of the non-autonomous and vulnerable members of society when they conflict with the wishes and interests of the autonomous members of society.

In summary, it is clear that competent patients should be free to make their own decisions regarding treatment, as discussed in the section on patient–carer relationships. The relationship between professionals and relatives should not include interference with the decision-making powers of competent patients, nor should professionals collude with relatives in impeding those powers.

3.3   The relatives as beneficiaries of professional care

Do health care professionals involved in palliative care have obligations to the relatives, and if so, what sort of benefits are they obliged to try to confer? For example, do they have obligations to further the health or emotional well-being of the relatives, or even to assist them in pursuit of other interests such as careers, financial affairs, holiday plans, etc.?

It is generally assumed in the context of palliative care (but not in most other aspects of health care) that professionals have obligations to benefit relatives. This assumption must at least be queried, and if accepted it must be justified.

We shall discuss the nature of possible obligations that professionals may have to relatives, and also the moral problems which arise when they appear to conflict with obligations to patients. In general, we consider that obligations to patients outweigh obligations to relatives. To put this point more strongly one might say that there can be obligations to relatives only when they are not outweighed by obligations to patients.

3.3.1 The obligation to prevent harm to the health of relatives

It seems to us illogical to suggest that an obligation on professionals to prevent harm to the health of relatives could ever be more compelling than their corresponding obligation to patients. It does seem plausible that professionals may have a greater obligation to prevent harm to the health of the relatives than to prevent similar harm to total strangers. However, the professionals' most compelling obligation is to further the health of the patient, because of the special relationship between them and also because of the great vulnerability of the patient. Occasionally, conflicts can occur between a professional's obligations to the patient and a possible obligation to prevent harm to the health of the relative.

In the preceding discussion on the relationship of professionals and relatives as co-carers of the patient we said that the health care team should not comply with the patient's wishes if to do so would result in physical harm to the relatives, and the examples given were those of an HIV positive patient and a patient who wished to be lifted by hand rather than by hoist. In these examples the obligations of confidentiality to the patient and to respect the patient's autonomy are outweighed by the obligation to prevent harm to the relatives.

A further and more common example of possible harm to relatives arises when highly dependent patients are at home. Sometimes, elderly relatives caring for a dying patient may become totally exhausted, even when the maximum available help has been provided at home. Professionals involved may then consider that the best way to prevent further harm to the relatives would be to move the patient to a specialist palliative care unit or hospital. However, if the patient is competent to make this decision then the patient's wishes must be respected, for it is not reasonable to force an unwilling patient to enter hospital (unless under the terms of the law relating to mental health). Of course in this case the professionals may well consider that their role is to make sure that the patient is informed regarding the exhaustion of the relatives. If the patient declines to move into institutional care then the professional's obligation to avoid harm to the relatives is subordinate to their obligation to respect the patient's choice to remain at home. When the patient is incompetent the moral situation is more difficult, as was explained earlier, because it may be impossible to ascertain what the wishes of the patient might have been in these circumstances, and the patient's wishes form part of the best interests judgement which the professionals must make on his or her behalf. In practice, incompetent patients are often moved into institutional care in this situation because professionals involved judge that such a move accords with their best interests, a judgement made by considering their medical good and likely wishes in the circumstances. It is important to make this judgement impartially on behalf of the patient, and then weigh it against the obligation to the relatives to avoid harm to them. If a conflict of obligations remains, then the likelihood and magnitude of serious harm to the relative and any possible harm to the patient will have to be weighed against each other. In general, we would consider that the obligation to prevent harm to the patient outweighs the obligation to prevent harm to the relatives, but we acknowledge that our position is contentious.

It should be noted that in stating that there is an obligation not to harm the health of relatives we are not saying that the relatives themselves become patients and so are owed the same obligations as patients, but rather that professionals have obligations not to cause harm and to prevent harm to the relatives as relatives.

3.3.2 *A possible obligation to give information to relatives*

The obligation to respect the autonomy of the patient with regard to information about the illness outweighs any possible obligation to give relatives information, apart from a few exceptional and rare circumstances where a significant risk of serious harm to the relatives justifies a breach of confidentiality. The example of the HIV positive patient receiving intimate care from relatives has already been described and is a situation where a breach of confidentiality would be justified.

Whilst the obligation to keep information confidential is generally known and acknowledged, and is clearly described in professional codes of conduct, it is surprising how often information is given to relatives without the patient's consent. One justification of this practice is that health care professionals may consider that it is in the patient's best interests to divulge the information, but this is definitely an explanation and not a justification. Another and more likely explanation is that professionals (and possibly relatives) may consider that there is some form of moral obligation to give relatives information about the patient's illness. For the purposes of discussion of such an obligation the circumstances of competent and incompetent patients are different in morally important ways and so should be considered separately.

Where the patient is competent to make decisions there seem to us no grounds for an obligation on professionals to divulge information to relatives. Patients can share as much information as they want with relatives, or may request that they be present at discussions with the health care team. Of course if patients request that professionals pass information direct to relatives then professionals respect their wishes in this regard. However, there seems no moral obligation to relatives to pass on information regarding competent patients, and indeed none is mentioned in professional codes of conduct.

In contrast, the situation with regard to incompetent patients is more complex. When relatives seek information the professional concerned should make a judgement as to whether the patient would have wanted the information passed on. Since in the vast majority of cases competent patients do want their close relatives informed about their illness, it will usually be the case that professionals will judge that the incompetent patient would want close relatives to be informed. This is especially true in the last few days of life when relatives benefit from explanation and reassurance. However, when patients have previously requested that a friend or relative should not be informed about the illness, then their wishes should continue to be respected when they are incompetent. This seems hard in some circumstances, such as occasionally arise when patients long estranged from a family member request that information should not be passed on to that person. It is much easier to divulge information in this case, but it is not justifiable and is a breach of confidentiality.

When health care professionals have to form a best interests judgement about treatment of an incompetent patient they should try to ascertain what the patient's wishes in the circumstances might be. In order to do this the circumstances must be explained to the relatives. This policy seems morally appropriate (so long as the patient had not previously stated that information should not be divulged to the relatives) because it accords with the patient's best interests.

In conclusion, we consider that there is no moral obligation to the relatives to divulge information. However, there are circumstances where an obligation to act in the patient's best interests requires professionals to divulge information, so long as the patient has not previously refused a request to do so. When patients are unconscious and dying it is humane to offer to relatives the explanations and reassurance which it may reasonably be considered the patient would have wished to be offered to them.

3.3.3   A possible obligation to offer 'counselling' to relatives

In the context of palliative care it is often said that relatives 'have a right' to counselling if they need or request it, regardless of the patient's wishes or needs. However, there are some moral difficulties with this view.

Firstly, 'counselling' in this case would normally entail giving explanations and answering questions about the nature of the illness, its likely progress, and the patient's needs in the future, all of which entails giving information about the patient's illness. As we have said, professionals giving any information regarding the patient's illness are subject to the obligations of confidentiality to the patient. It is easy, but not justifiable, when talking to relatives and answering their queries to give them more information about the illness and its likely progress than the patient possesses. Health care professionals have a natural desire to assist the relatives by answering their questions, and it can be difficult to remember that the patient is the person primarily entitled to information about the illness, and that this information should be passed on only with the competent patient's consent.

Secondly, psychological support requires time, and since time is often the most scarce and valuable resource the health care team possesses, it must be apportioned justly. It is widely recognized that the psychological trauma of a terminal illness may be as great for relatives as it is for patients, for example when the patient is a much loved spouse or child. It is therefore understandable that health care workers often consider that their obligation to relatives to provide psychological support is as great as their corresponding obligation to patients. Yet there must be limits to our obligations towards relatives in this respect. We would argue that the time used for psychological support of relatives should not be disproportionate to that which is needed for essential medical and nursing treatment (and psychological support) of patients. It is not uncommon in the context of palliative care for relatives requesting emotional support to take up so much of the health professionals' time that patients actually receive less attention than the relatives. As patients become more unwell and tired they tend to require more nursing care but often less time for discussion of the progress of the illness or treatment options. Whilst they frequently have less energy for long conversations, their comfort is largely dependent on excellent unhurried care and symptom control, and they are extremely vulnerable to constraints on the resource of professional time. It is easy and understandable for professionals to give in to the relatives' expectation of considerable time for their psychological support, but it is not morally justifiable to do so if, in consequence, patients are deprived of the time essential for their physical and psychological comfort. It is always easier for professionals to grant the wishes of the most assertive claimant, and at the end of the patient's life the most assertive claimant is often a relative. In this situation we need to remind ourselves that when this conflict arises, our obligations to meet the patient's needs outweigh our obligations to 'counsel' the relatives.

3.3.4 A possible obligation to relieve the relatives' psychological suffering

It is sometimes claimed that there is an obligation to relieve the relatives' psychological suffering where possible, but if this is so then obviously conflicts of obligation will arise because there is clearly an obligation to minimize or relieve the patient's psychological suffering. Some people would argue that the obligation to benefit relatives in this way is more compelling than the corresponding obligation to patients. Two arguments can be produced for this view.

Firstly, it may be said that the maximum relief of suffering and enhancement of well-being of all concerned is achieved by benefiting the relatives psychologically rather than acting in the patient's best interests if there is a case of conflict. This conclusion is reached by those who consider that the most important moral aim is to achieve the best consequences in terms of relief of overall suffering and enhancement of well-being. They point out that in the context of palliative care the relatives are going to live for much longer than the patient, so whilst the patient stands to benefit physically and psychologically for only a short time, the relatives will benefit psychologically for a much longer time and in bereavement may suffer less physical morbidity. Thus if the relatives' welfare is enhanced by granting their wishes, the overall well-being of all people concerned is increased more than if the patient's well-being were prioritized. It is further argued that if there is harm to the patient this is of relatively short duration compared with the harm which may be done to a relative who may live for many years with residual psychological trauma. According to this view the wishes and well-being of patients would be habitually overridden by the wishes and well-being of relatives, on the grounds that as the relatives live longer greater aggregate benefit would be derived. The consequences to patients of this utilitarian argument are disastrous. For example, patients would be admitted to hospitals and specialist palliative care units against their best interests for the psychological benefit of relatives.

A second argument for benefiting the relatives as much or more than patients is that they may litigate against health care professionals if their wishes are not granted. We have already pointed out that litigation is very unpleasant for professionals, since it is an attack on their personal competence, integrity, and reputation, and it consumes resources of time and money which are often diverted from patient care. Whilst this is an explanation of why professionals may decide to benefit relatives psychologically to the detriment of the patient's care, it is not a moral justification for doing so. Health professionals may be tempted to instigate treatment, such as artificial nutrition or hydration which is not in the dying and incompetent patient's interests, in order to give psychological benefit to relatives who are unable to accept that such treatment is invasive and no longer beneficial. We consider that it is not morally acceptable to provide inappropriate treatment in order to benefit the relatives psychologically and so minimize the possibility of litigation.

We do not consider that either of the above weak arguments justifies a policy of permitting a possible obligation to benefit relatives psychologically to override our obligations to benefit patients. However, it should be noted that even if one considers that the obligation to benefit relatives psychologically is as compelling as the corresponding obligation to patients, a physical harm to patients cannot be justified by a psychological benefit to relatives. Consider the common situation where we have to balance the conflicting needs of patients in our care but where we recognize that we have an equal obligation to each one. Due to lack of resources we often have to limit the benefit to one in order to achieve a benefit for another. But we do not consider it morally justifiable to inflict actual medical harm on one patient for the benefit of another. So even if our obligation to benefit relatives equals that to patients we are not justified in inflicting harm on the patient in order to benefit the relatives, either physically or psychologically. Thus although it is often tempting and seems easier to give inappropriate and possibly harmful treatment to a patient in order to meet a perceived obligation to benefit the relatives, it is not morally justifiable to do so.

Having rejected these weak arguments for giving relatives priority, we shall now argue that the obligation to benefit relatives psychologically is less compelling than that to benefit patients for the following reasons.

Firstly, patients in the context of palliative care are often weak and tired if not frankly exhausted. They often lack the energy to assert their point of view and may tend to take the line of least resistance. Where their interests conflict with those of relatives, they are the least able party to assert their views and argue their own case. If health care professionals consider that their obligation to benefit relatives is as strong as that to benefit patients, and the views of patients are usually put forward much less assertively because of their weakness, then professionals will tend to act in favour of relatives' interests and at the expense of patients' interests. Patients will then no longer be able to trust in the professionals' commitment to their good, and the fundamental basis of the relationship between patient and professional will be seriously jeopardized or lost.

Secondly, we believe that the purpose of health care is to benefit patients, in terms of prolonging life and alleviating suffering due to disease. The aim of health care is neither to benefit relatives of patients nor to maximize the aggregate general well-being of members of society.

Thus we would conclude that any obligation to benefit relatives must be less compelling than that to benefit patients, firstly in order to achieve the aims of health care, and secondly in order to prevent the injustice of overriding the interests of less autonomous patients by their more autonomous relatives.

It may be argued that the interests of relatives and patients are inextricably intertwined, especially when the relationship is very close, such as between parents and children or spouses. But the moral problems which arise in palliative care commonly concern conflict between the interests of relatives and patients, and professionals are occasionally faced with an unresolvable dilemma where they must choose between serving the interests of either the patient or the relative. This occurs particularly regarding the place of care, when it is not uncommon for patients to wish to remain in their home, but for relatives to feel that they do not want to shoulder the physical and psychological burdens of caring for the patient there.

In weighing up possible competing obligations to relatives and patients in particular circumstances, the magnitude of the benefits concerned is obviously of moral relevance. For example, it is generally justifiable (and indeed morally required) to forgo a minor benefit to a relative for the sake of a major benefit to the patient, especially if one considers, as we do, that one has a stronger obligation to benefit patients than relatives. It may be justifiable to forego a minor benefit to a patient for the sake of a major benefit to a relative. However, it must be remembered that infliction of actual harm on either party by the health care professional in order to achieve a benefit for the other cannot be justified. This applies particularly where the infliction of a medical harm to a patient for sake of a benefit to relatives is concerned.

It is important that this latter principle is upheld by clinicians in practice. As we have said, futile or harmful treatments are sometimes given to patients at the request of relatives and with the intention of benefiting the relatives psychologically. For example, if relatives request that a terminally ill patient be resuscitated at the end of life when the medical team are certain from the clinical facts and published evidence that the attempt will not succeed, it is the practice in some medical cultures to pretend to resuscitate the patient by using inadequate techniques. It is argued that this lessens the harm to the patient whilst still 'benefiting' the relatives. It may also be argued that it is not possible to harm someone who is going to die anyway—but if this view is accepted then all harm to terminally ill patients would be considered morally irrelevant, a conclusion which is clearly wrong. In reality, a failed resuscitation attempt, even a false one, is not a peaceful or dignified death for the patient and is certainly a harm.

Further harms ensue in that health care professionals in training come to regard this practice as acceptable, and come to believe that inflicting harmful treatments on patients for the sake of relatives is morally justified. They further come to believe that deceiving relatives is morally justified by the suggested benefit of their psychological well-being, although the true motivation of health care professionals in this situation may well be the avoidance of conflict and the threat of litigation.

Whatever the relative–professional relationship should be, it should not be one of deceit, for this is morally destructive of professionals and disrespectful to relatives. Nor should it be one where the prevailing element from the professional's perspective is fear of confrontation, conflict, and litigation, for a relationship based on these elements is coercive to professionals and severely impedes their clinical judgement and decision making. The patients' good is unlikely to be served by such a climate of fear, and indeed patients are likely to be harmed.

3.3.5   The obligation to respect the relatives' autonomy

The concept of respect for autonomy often causes confusion when applied to relatives. Its meaning in the context of patient care was clarified in the chapter on the patient–carer relationship. In that context health care professionals consider that the principle of respect for the patient's autonomy means that they have an obligation to assist patients to attain their own reasonable goals with regard to treatment and the place and manner of their remaining life and death.

We should also consider what respect for the autonomy of relatives might entail. Since autonomy is self-rule, it relates to the conduct of the individual's own life, not that of another. So respecting the autonomy of relatives entails permitting them to make choices about the conduct of their own lives. It does not entail assisting them to make choices about the conduct of the patient's life.

In particular, it should be noted that respect for the autonomy of one person cannot entail assisting that person to attain a goal which is harmful to another human being. This is especially the case where one has special role obligations to that other human being, as health care professionals do to their patients. Therefore, respect for the autonomy of relatives cannot entail assisting them to achieve goals which result in harm to the patient, and so any obligation to respect the autonomy of the relatives must be limited. It must be remembered that respect for the autonomy of patients is also limited. It requires that we encourage their involvement in decision making and do not override their informed refusal of treatment, even if their relatives would prefer them to undergo the refused option. It also requires that at each stage of the illness we endeavour to enable patients to be cared for in the place of their choice and that we do not remove them from their homes against their will. But at the same time patients cannot demand inappropriate treatment from health care professionals, nor can they demand from relatives a level of care which those relatives do not feel able to provide. When conflicts of interest occur between relatives and patients, and health care professionals consider that they have an obligation to respect the autonomy of both, it is helpful to be reminded of the limits of such respect in each case.

Increasingly frequently it is argued that respect for autonomy is the overriding principle in health care, and that one should respect the autonomy of whoever has it, whether they be relative or patient. A similar argument is presented by those who believe that the function of health care is to maximize autonomy (as opposed to relieving suffering or prolonging life). According to this view, autonomy can be maximized most effectively by concentrating on the relatives, because patients may already have compromised and decreasing autonomy. Thus those who believe that the function of health care is to maximize autonomy are likely to strive to enhance the autonomy of relatives by granting their wishes as opposed to the wishes of patients whose status with regard to autonomy is frequently declining. But this is a weak argument which has disastrous consequences. For in practice it results in harming or failing to benefit vulnerable, less assertive, and less autonomous people like patients, to whom we have special obligations, for the sake of respecting and enhancing the autonomy of relatives. We deal in more detail with the principle of respect for autonomy in Chapter 13, p. 278.

3.4 Attitudes in the relative–professional relationship

As in the patient–carer relationship, relatives must be able to trust that professionals are committed to the patient's welfare. They must also be able to trust in the honesty and integrity of professionals, and any attempts by professionals to mislead relatives or patients undermine that essential trust.

In a climate of increasing litigation there is a tendency for an attitude of anxiety and sometimes fear to enter the relationship between health carers and relatives. This is ultimately detrimental to patient care. Health care professionals require the quality of moral courage to remain committed to the patient's good, and in particular to refuse to give harmful treatments to patients because of misguided requests from relatives.

An attitude of benevolence towards relatives is appropriate on behalf of health care professionals, who should strive to prevent harm to them and to benefit them, within the necessary constraints of the requirement to benefit patients.

Decisions involving conflicts of interest between relatives and patients are always difficult. If such conflicts cannot be resolved and a choice must be made, then professionals should analyse the problem in terms of their overriding obligations in the particular circumstances. There may be no ideal solution, and more than one course of action may be morally justifiable.

3.5 Conclusions

1. When relatives are caring for patients, health care professionals should try to prevent relatives and patients from

harming each other, whilst recognizing the limits to professional intervention in the home.

2. Parents may consent to or refuse treatment on behalf of their child, but the role of relatives of incompetent adult patients is to inform professional carers of the patient's previously expressed wishes, goals, and values.

3. Since it is only in the context of the patient–carer relationship that the professional encounters the relatives, and commitment to the patient's good is the foundation of the patient–carer relationship, obligations to the patient will take precedence over any obligation to benefit the relatives.

4. Obligations of confidentiality apply when divulging information about the patient to relatives. The professional obligation is primarily to inform the patient; professionals should not withhold information from patients because relatives request that they should do so.

5. Since autonomy is self-rule, the autonomy of relatives relates to the conduct of their own lives, not that of the patient. Professionals should respect the autonomy of relatives with regard to the conduct of their own lives, but they are not obliged to accede to the relatives' wishes with regard to the treatment of adult patients. Thus professionals should not provide clinically inappropriate treatment to patients at the request of relatives.

4

Teamwork

A *monologue is not a decision.*
Clement Attlee, *A Prime Minister Remembers*, Ch. 7 (1961)

Democracy means government by discussion, but it is only effective if you can stop people talking.
Clement Attlee, *Speech at Oxford*, 14 June 1957

4.1 Why do we work in teams?

The concept of the multidisciplinary team has always been central to the philosophy of palliative care. The knowledge and skills of many health care professionals are essential if the intrinsic and extrinsic aims of palliative care are to be met. Specialist palliative care teams in in-patient units tend to consist of a relatively small and stable nucleus of professionals, and patients are referred to the whole team for care. Such teams are often based in hospices or dedicated wards in NHS hospitals where the staff form a discrete group who work closely together, whilst liaising with primary care teams and other hospital colleagues involved in the patient's care.

The situation in any ward in the general hospital setting is not dissimilar. Medical, nursing, and other staff tend to work together in stable groups. Although management structures and lines of accountability are separate for each discipline, clinical patient care is undertaken by the multidisciplinary group.

Primary care teams are also relatively stable, comprising mainly medical, nursing, and administrative staff, but increasingly other professionals such as physiotherapists and clinical psychologists are employed on a sessional basis so that they too become part of the group.

Thus from a managerial point of view a multidisciplinary team structure is established in specialist palliative care units, in general hospitals, and in the community. Health care is delivered through this structure which essentially comprises nuclei of multiprofessional expertise. Current health care policy is very much team-focused.

Specialists in palliative care have become increasingly committed
to the idea of teamwork, and to the establishment and preservation
of this stable nucleus of carers, to such an extent that the term
'multidisciplinary team' has almost become a cliché. In palliative
care units the professional team is constituted before the patient is
encountered, and guidelines state that doctors, nurses, social workers,
physiotherapists, chaplains, and so on are all essential members.
Thus the professionals are gathered into a working group which has
clear boundaries in a philosophical and managerial sense. Over the
course of time the group becomes tightly bonded as well as clearly
defined.

The team exists to fulfil its aims in palliative care. Each member
has a distinctive and important role to play, and is considered
essential to the fulfilment of the team aims. One member has a
predominant leadership role, but leadership will vary according to
the circumstances and immediate goals. The team is relatively stable,
and seeks to assess or measure its performance.

Moral justification for our support of the nuclear team in specialist palliative care might be based on its consequences in three areas—
individual patient care, the working environment for carers, and
cost-effectiveness. We might also consider that working together in a
stable group towards agreed goals may be 'good in itself', in that it
contributes to our understanding of ourselves as social beings. These
advantages require consideration and then comparison with the
practical and moral difficulties which can occur in teamwork and
which threaten the achievement of the aims of the team.

Effective and compassionate patient care is the goal of all involved
in palliative care, and teamwork can contribute to this by encouraging good communication between professionals so that the skills
and knowledge needed can be obtained from members of the team
who pool their expertise when considering clinical problems. The
stability of the team ensures that repetitive transfer of information to
continuously changing members is avoided and, since the team is
relatively small, confidential information is less widely disseminated
than would be the case if frequently changing carers were involved.
Team members inevitably teach each other in the course of discussion and are stimulated to improve and enlarge the knowledge base
of palliative care. In a successful team morale is good and members
support and encourage each other so that the highest possible standards of care are achieved, even when circumstances are difficult.

Many professionals also feel that a team environment is in their interests. It is more enjoyable to work in a happy group than alone, and humour especially is a great source of pleasure. More importantly, the mutual support from other team members helps carers to cope with the considerable emotional stresses of working with patients who are terminally ill. The constant impact of sadness and loss, plus other stresses such as pressure of time and the demands of management, all contribute to the much discussed phenomenon of 'burn out' or emotional exhaustion in professional carers. Team members are usually supportive of each other and their ability to work cooperatively and flexibly means that difficult problems and peaks in workload can be shared. Physical and emotional exhaustion then becomes less likely. Similarly, the example of skilled and compassionate care by other team members inspires individuals to work effectively beyond the point at which they might otherwise lapse into cynicism or despondency. Listening to the views of others also helps carers to see clinical problems from different points of view, and indirectly promotes self-development which in turn leads to a greater sense of fulfilment at work and enjoyment from life in general. Lastly, team members learn to trust each other, and realize that no-one is indispensable. Carers can then leave at the end of a shift and relax mentally, confident that others will care effectively for the patient. This helps to prevent emotional exhaustion. Moreover, as trust and confidence are established, humility tends to follow as we appreciate the strengths of colleagues.

The nuclear team may be the most cost-effective way of delivering palliative care, ensuring that a given fund of money and professional expertise is used to the maximum benefit. Since our methods of measuring outcomes in palliative care are fairly primitive at present, it would be very difficult to prove that the team as described is the most cost-effective way of providing such care. Financial costs can be counted relatively easily, but reliable and valid measures of effectiveness are difficult to establish.

Finally, it could be said that apart from its consequences teamwork may be morally good in itself. There may be intrinsic moral value in working together instead of as individuals whose activities are coordinated by a manager. Such a value might be based on our understanding of ourselves as primarily social beings who naturally live and work in communities. The achievement of working together successfully towards the goal of palliative care strengthens our bonds

to each other, and forces us to acknowledge our mutual inter-
dependence whilst making it apparent that this very interdepen-
dence can be used to the advantage of all. Working together as a
team may be a morally important goal for human beings, apart from
its beneficial consequences for patients, professionals, and society.

These reasons together may seem to provide an overwhelming
argument for the maintenance of stable nuclei of professional expertise in palliative care, whether based in the community, hospice, or
hospital setting, but there are problems inherent in teamwork, and so
moral justification for our support for this model of care must rest
on a balance of good over harm to the patients, carers, and society. It
should be noted that the problems described below will be likely in
any close-knit nuclear health care team.

4.2   Common problems in specialist palliative care teams

We have said that there are problems inherent in teamwork, and
professionals involved for any length of time in a specialist palliative
care team will experience some of them. Serious problems compromise the ability of the team to achieve its aim, and ultimately patient
care suffers. Carers may also be harmed in various ways, and partners
and families of patients and carers may suffer indirectly. Society is
adversely affected if resources are not best used, or if care becomes
less effective and therefore public anxiety about terminal illness
increases.

Thus any major problem in the team has moral implications. Since
the initial development of specialist palliative care teams, which began
as groups of dedicated professionals working together in hospices
which were usually charitably funded, some problems have emerged
which do have serious practical and therefore moral consequences.

The close-knit nature of the team, which can become intellectually
'cosy', may discourage its members from challenging its goals and
values because it is easier and more comfortable not to threaten the
attractive assumptions which the team may be making. Intellectual
cosiness is really the result of a shared belief system which members
of the team have become reluctant to question or re-examine. In
palliative care such shared beliefs might include the idea that we
have obligations to benefit the relatives as well as the patient.
Practices and policies may also become established because of shared

beliefs and assumptions. For example, it m
bed empty overnight after a death in order
adjust to the loss; if, however, this policy
to other patients who urgently need the be
to question the policy. This may be difficult
is attractive to carers and probably to patier
ist unit. Established policies can become di
many team members adhere to them. This can lead to an insular
attitude within the team, and this encourages narrow-mindedness
which tends to cause further isolation from the outside world of
health care and the community. Team attitudes may inappropriately
remain stationary while the rest of the world moves on. Attitudes do
not necessarily have to change, but it must be possible to question
them. A team (and its values) is not a fixed entity cast in stone; it
must be capable of self-review and change.

Similarly, individuals within the team may become so dependent
on the security it gives them that they cease to think for themselves,
losing their capacity for independent-mindedness which is important
in personal development. As professionals we do have a duty to
develop ourselves, not just to enable us to be more compassionate
and understanding carers but also to enable us to 'be all we can be'
and in so doing gain fulfilment from life in general.

Sometimes the phenomenon of 'scapegoating' occurs in palliative
care teams. In this situation an unpopular person in the team comes
to be blamed unjustly for all ills, with an underlying assumption that
without them all would be well and the team would function
perfectly. Life may be made so uncomfortable for this member that
he or she may leave the team, their contribution to difficulties having
been unjustifiably magnified. This may occur when the team is not
dealing with internal or external problems successfully, and is
seeking someone to blame, in the way that human beings so often
do! The personal cost to this member in trauma resulting from
feelings of failure, rejection, and anger can be very high. The team
should not seek escape from its difficulties or exoneration from its
failings by sacrificing the welfare of individual members by unjustly
attributing blame to them. In fact, other problems will inevitably
arise, because there is no such thing as an internally perfect team, or
one without external difficulties. The solution to such problems does
not lie in eliminating members if they are not truly the cause of the
difficulties.

ther conflicts between team members such as leadership battles, disagreements over care policies or decisions, and distribution of labour and rewards can all fester and become magnified in the microcosm of a close-knit palliative care team. This leads to unhappiness which can be so severe as to detract from the ability of staff to do their job well, and gossiping about the problems can consume valuable time that should be devoted to patient care. Simmering anger and feelings of impotence to alter the situation consume energy and cause misery. Such conflicts are frequently destructive of more than one team member, and can lead to less than optimal functioning of the whole team.

In contrast, it is possible to focus so much energy on the welfare of the team that a form of introversion may result, and the interests of the team may be given a higher priority than patient care. There is a delicate balance between the priorities of patient care and maintaining morale and integration in the team. If we feel that the latter has to be maintained in order to ensure the former, then logically they become equal in importance. But we know that good morale and a happy working atmosphere will not alone guarantee good palliative care—many other factors are essential. Moreover, the ultimate goal of palliative care is the patient's good, not the welfare of the team and its members.

A difficult debate surrounds the issue of how much harm, if any, can justifiably be inflicted on professional carers for the sake of the patient. It must depend, as always, on the circumstances, and some harms such as the emotional trauma of witnessing a fatal haematemesis or physical exhaustion after an exceptionally heavy shift are unavoidable. Justification of any harms which are preventable rests on many morally relevant factors such as the balance of harms and benefits to carer and patient, and the willingness of the carer to act altruistically. In general terms one might say that if staff wish to care for the patient 'beyond the reasonable calls of duty', then their autonomy should be respected and they should be allowed to do so, unless other members feel that unacceptable harm is consistently being done to them or to the rest of the team in the process.

In contrast, if the tasks of palliative care team cannot usually be met within the bounds of the professionals' duty, and constant self-sacrifice is required, then clearly the staffing level or structure is inappropriate to the expectation of performance. In this case some agreed limits have to be placed on workload after wide consultation between users and providers of the service, and/or the level of staffing should be increased. It will exceptionally happen that patients' needs can be met only by self-sacrifice on behalf of the staff, but ideally when this situation arises it should be tackled following a team discussion to ensure fair distribution of extra labour amongst those who are willing and able to shoulder the burden. The quality of routine care for patients should not rely on altruistic or supererogatory acts (those beyond the call of duty) on behalf of carers. Management has a duty to safeguard workers as far as possible against the harms of physical and emotional exhaustion due to overwork.

It remains difficult to justify denying patients a reasonable standard of care in order to avoid harming the staff; where there is good management and a mature team this conflict of interests should be prevented.

The assumption that working the staff ever harder will achieve or sustain high quality care is at least questionable and in our view is probably false. Physical and emotional exhaustion, disillusionment and perhaps cynicism about management must logically lead to rising sickness levels, a higher turnover of staff, and a constant feeling of stress and low morale. This climate is unlikely to lead to high quality patient care. Thus if excessive workload does not lead to high quality care and instead contributes to less than satisfactory care, then management actually has a responsibility to keep the workload in reasonable proportion to the human resources available, even if rationing of the service is required. Therefore, management has an obligation to place limits on workload for the sake of patients, quite apart from their obligations not to exploit or harm the staff.

Sometimes professional carers use the team to meet too many personal aims or inappropriate personal aims, such as the need for affection, self-esteem, company, etc. Such aims should not be met exclusively through the professional's role in palliative care. If they are, then the welfare of the carer is dependent to an excessive degree on their happiness and success at work. The danger is that the aim of patient care can become subordinate to the need to satisfy personal needs and achieve personal goals. What may appear as complete devotion to the professional role may actually be an excuse not to meet the challenges of making deep personal relationships outside the team. If a team member rarely goes home on time and seems totally absorbed in the job, then it is possible that few personal aims or needs are being met outside the work environment. This is likely to lead to problems at work which in turn comes to assume overwhelming importance in that person's life.

It may be difficult to define the extent to which the drive to meet personal needs through work is either cause or effect—does the professional enter palliative care because he or she consciously or unconsciously sees it as a way to meet personal needs, or does the job come to occupy so much time and emotional energy that no resources remain to develop a life outside the workplace? The latter situation, as we have said, constitutes a harm to the carer which is not morally justifiable. In general, however, it is not inappropriate to meet some personal needs and achieve some personal aims through palliative care, providing that the welfare of patients, lay carers, and other team members is not compromised.

In contrast, many teams are so comfortable, stimulating, and humorous to work in that time can be wasted by members enjoying each other's company and talking too much about matters not relevant to the task. It also has to be said that in palliative care light relief from emotionally charged situations is essential. The correct balance between fun and work can be difficult to strike.

If the nuclear team is very isolated from other professionals, communication with other teams is not encouraged, and such isolation can easily foster a climate of disrespect and even potential aggression and conflict with other teams, particularly when resources or philosophies of care are at stake. For example, tension can easily develop between specialist palliative care teams and oncology teams, or between acute medical teams and those caring for the elderly. These tensions arise because the teams view similar clinical situations in slightly different ways, and each team considers that their own view of optimum patient care is the most appropriate. Isolation tends to perpetuate prejudices and prevents team members from trying to see or being able to appreciate alternative points of view. If tensions develop into conflicts they have a tendency to be destructive of all teams involved, rather than having a constructive effect.

All of these potential harms exist because no human being is morally perfect, and so no team is perfect. Teamwork in palliative care still yields a balance of good over harm if the problems listed above can be avoided, solved, or at least minimized. Since the origin of the problems is human nature itself, none of them can be eliminated altogether, and so the efforts of all team members are required to find solutions and to minimize the harms incurred by all concerned.

It can be difficult for professionals specializing in palliative care to keep internal team problems in perspective. This happens because the small stable nucleus of highly motivated carers becomes a microcosm in which intense feelings are likely because of the emotionally charged nature of the work. Quite simply, 'so much seems to be at stake'. The last days and weeks of life always seem so precious because time is limited, and conflicts over care plans can easily develop into power struggles between team members. Feelings of frustration are intense if staff feel they are not able to do the job well; they know there is not going to be a 'second chance' to get things right if mistakes are made or opportunities lost. The close-knit nature of the typical hospice or NHS specialist palliative care team, which may function under conditions of relative philosophical and geographical isolation from other health carers, tends to exacerbate many of the problems by effectively blowing them out of proportion and discouraging the dissipation of intense emotions. In addition, there may be no access to help from outside when serious difficulties arise, or the team may be reluctant to use such help because members see it as a threat to the entire philosophy, standards, and integrity of the team, or feel as a matter of pride and loyalty that they should always solve internal problems internally.

Unfortunately, this model of a team, which could be described as tightly bonded and bounded in a managerial and philosophical sense, or as 'teamwork narrowly conceived', is the current model for any specialist palliative care team providing the highest level of multidisciplinary expertise. We know that this model can be effective when dealing with the most difficult clinical problems precisely because of the high degree of staff motivation, but it has built-in problems and the human costs of the care it provides can be high.

4.3 Patient-centred or management-centred teams

An idea of 'teamwork broadly conceived' might enable us to preserve the major advantages of working together whilst avoiding or minimizing the problems. A concept of a team which is less tightly bonded and bounded may be appropriate. It helps at this point to question some of our initial assumptions.

The patient wants and needs competent compassionate care from all the professionals whose skills and knowledge are necessary. It is obviously helpful if those carers communicate with each other so that the patient is spared unnecessary repetition of information. On the other hand, most patients want confidentiality to be preserved as far as possible, and so want personal information shared between the minimum number of staff, divulged only on a 'need to know' basis.

Patients may not have a narrow concept of a team, but are more likely to see themselves as drawing on a pool of professionals with whom they can work flexibly and imaginatively to solve problems. From the patient's perspective, the team comprises all those involved in their care. It is not a fixed structure as it may be in the minds of members of the palliative care team and health care managers. Moreover, the patient will want to be included as a key member of the decision-making team, and relatives form a vital part of the caring team especially when the patient is at home. Thus it is likely that the concept of the nuclear team in a managerial sense is owned much more by the professionals themselves than by the patient. Indeed we would argue that the patient's perspective may more accurately reflect what should happen in practice.

Whilst the ward staff of geographically isolated specialist palliative care units may work almost exclusively as crucial members of nuclear teams, doctors and nurses working in the community or general hospital setting, and doctors based in hospices but with an educational and advisory role outside the hospice are in fact members of many interlocking teams both large and small. In these teams they play varying roles, as leaders or followers, central key-players or peripheral members, as managers or front-line workers. Doctors are often members of a ward team, a home care team working in the community, a hospital advisory service, an educational team, and the wider team of the local and also the national health service. Specialist palliative care nurses are similarly members of many teams. Thus the 'nuclear team' approach to palliative care may differ from what actually happens.

Managers have an increasing role to play in health care. Whilst most staff involved in clinical care consider that the role of managers is to provide clinical staff with the environment and resources to do their job well, some managers regard themselves as outside the large team, and function in a 'controlling' rather than a 'facilitating' capacity. This is less likely if clinical staff try to involve managers as much as possible in clinical activities and service plans, so that problems are seen by both sides as difficulties which need to be resolved together. Involvement with others tends to draw us close together. Managers, like carers, have professional and personal aims at stake in their jobs. Despite the difficulties, clinical staff should treat them with the same regard and respect that they grant each other. It is expedient and also morally appropriate to involve managers as members of the wider team.

From the patient's perspective what actually matters is that all those needed, including relatives and friends involved in care, are seen to be able and willing to work together flexibly. This is most likely if palliative care specialists regard themselves not only as members of many interlocking teams in a managerial sense, but also as an important member of each small and flexibly constituted team of people orientated around each patient.

This broader view of teamwork helps to minimize isolation and narrow-mindedness, and prevents personal conflicts from becoming magnified in importance. Constant involvement in many patient-centred teams inevitably leads to learning, and helps all carers to keep problems in perspective and set reasonable goals. When we witness difficulties in other teams in which we play a minor role, we may come to understand those same difficulties from a different point of view when they arise in the teams in which we play a major role. We can achieve this general broad-mindedness without losing our philosophy of care. In fact, specialists in palliative care will be challenged to re-examine their values and practices continually, so that they remain appropriate in the changing circumstances of palliative care as it evolves.

In conclusion we may say that whilst there are stable multi-professional teams organized from a managerial perspective, the team which should actually be most important in palliative care comprises all individuals actually involved in the care of each particular patient. Such a team is necessarily different for each patient, especially in the community setting. Patient care should not be bounded by the limits set by the managerial organization of hospice, hospital, or primary care teams. Rather it should be orientated around and towards the patient and be delivered by input from members of many interlocking teams. This ideal accords with the philosophy of palliative care, and minimizes some of the problems inherent in the nuclear team approach.

4.4 Working in a patient-centred team

Much time has been devoted to the study of how teams work by those involved in management and industry. Such studies usually presuppose that the team is relatively stable, and that not all the members are necessarily professionals in their own right. They also stress the role of leader whose task 'involves focusing the efforts of a group of people towards a common goal and enabling them to work together as a team' (Adair 1987). It then follows that the leader's tasks are threefold; to achieve the task, to build and maintain the team, and to develop individuals in the team to their maximum potential. It is also sometimes said that the leader should also strive to attain ever greater performance from the team, but this seems irrational since there are limits to everyone's physical and mental resources, and it seems wrong to insinuate that whatever the team achieves it will never be good enough.

This typical management model of a team may be appropriate and useful to health service managers, especially in the market economy model of health care, but it is not appropriate in palliative care where a patient-centred team is morally and practically preferable. Here the decision-making team comprises a changing and flexible group of professionals together with the patient, and often the relatives if they are involved in care or if the patient is incompetent. Such a team is not one constituted by management, and standard approaches to teambuilding including leadership, concepts of responsibility, and ways of dealing with conflict and so on are not necessarily appropriate.

A typical patient-centred team in the community setting might comprise the patient and relatives, the general practitioner and community nurses, plus other practice staff such as receptionists and paramedical staff, plus any hospital or specialist palliative care staff who may be involved in the patient's care at home at the request of the general practitioner. In this situation the general practitioner is held responsible for the patient's care, but this care and associated decisions involve all members of the team.

In contrast, the hospital or specialist palliative care unit team comprises the patient (and perhaps the relatives), a consultant and supporting medical staff, nursing staff managed in a hierarchical structure, paramedical and ancillary staff, and often the general practitioner and community nurses at the interface of in-patient and community care. Hospital management staff are involved peripherally in trying to provide clinical staff with whatever is needed to do the job well.

The question of leadership arises in both settings, as does the related question of responsibility for the way decisions are made and for the outcomes which result directly from those decisions. Unlike the management model there is no imperative to build a strong and lasting team, only to enable all to work together to attain the patient's good. In palliative care the patient-centred team exists only to further the patient's good. Since this aim is intrinsic to professionals involved in palliative care, no other motivation from outside the team is necessary. A leader is therefore not required to build or maintain the team, or to motivate patient and professionals, or to be responsible for the personal development of professionals or patients. Is there then a professional leadership role in the patient-centred team? It seems that in the managerial sense there is not. Different members of the team will have primary responsibility for some decisions by virtue of their professional expertise, and may lead in the context of those decisions, but a general leadership role is not necessary. A model of professional partnership is more appropriate. We acknowledge that in a managerially constituted team, such as a hospital, specialist palliative care unit, or primary care team, a leadership role as described does exist, but it is not part of front-line palliative care at the level of individual clinical decisions.

Moral and legal responsibility for the way in which decisions are made and for the outcomes which result from those decisions are complex issues which involve concepts of collective responsibility. In previous chapters we have concentrated on the simpler topic of individual responsibility. In the clinical situation, where several professionals and the patient (perhaps with some input from relatives) all contribute to management decisions, the question arises as to whether a 'team' can actually make a decision at all, let alone take moral and legal responsibility for it. Whilst acknowledging that this presents philosophical and practical difficulties, it seems logical to argue that if the team is the unit of provision of palliative care, then that team should also be responsible for making management decisions. The care plan for a patient is derived through the decision-making process, which in turn leads to outcomes. If the team makes the decisions, then the team must in some way be responsible for the way they are made and for outcomes which result.

4.5   Collective responsibility

Is collective responsibility a reality, and if so what exactly does it mean when applied to teamwork in palliative care? Is it just a convenient fiction to support the desirable concept of teamwork ? If there is no such thing as true collective responsibility, then it might be suggested that there is no such thing as truly collaborative decision making by the team. There are several different ways of considering the possibility of collective responsibility.

In the first sense, a number of professionals who are all individually responsible for their practice operate together as a group. This would be the situation in a team of specialist palliative care nurses working in the community where each has a personal case-load, even though they may provide cross-cover for patient care at weekends and during annual leave. They are each responsible for their own actions as individuals, but together they have *aggregate responsibility* for the entire group of patients they serve. This is simply the sum of individual responsibility.

In a second sense, a group of health care workers could all contribute to a discussion on patient management, but the final responsibility for selection of the care options offered lies with a single member of the team, very often the consultant or general practitioner. If the clinical problem is primarily related to nursing care, then the community nurse or ward sister will ultimately make the decision after consultation with colleagues, and will be accountable for it. Each professional member of the team is responsible for their contribution to the discussion, but final accountability rests with one member who is frequently the leader in a managerial sense. This could be termed *hierarchical responsibility* and in reality it is the commonest form of collective responsibility in palliative care today. But it is not a true form of collective responsibility.

At the beginning of this chapter it was stated that the aims of palliative care require the diverse knowledge and skills of many professions and the achievement of the patient's total good is dependent on their collective efforts. In this sense responsibility for the success of palliative care must be truly collective, since none of the professionals acts alone: each is dependent on the others. This third concept is one of true collective responsibility for the patient's total good. It could be termed *multiprofessional responsibility*. If it is true collective responsibility then the team as a whole is liable to praise or blame for the actions done in its name.

This concept of true collective responsibility would require that the professionals offering treatments or suggesting care plans to the patient should do so after a consensus decision has been made. Since individual and professional values do vary, the achievement of consensus would sometimes require a degree of compromise on behalf of individuals. All are required to cooperate in the final course of action, so ideally all must 'own' the decision. This is most likely to be the case if decisions are reached by consensus. In achieving this consensus we are not suggesting that individuals should compromise their own consciences, although this might rarely be necessary. Rather we suggest that a conscientious compromise is reached which all the professionals feel they can support both ideologically and practically. Rarely in palliative care such a conscientious compromise does not appear possible to one or more team members, and then a situation of moral conflict within the team has to be resolved.

4.6 Moral conflict in the team

Whilst an increasing number of decisions relating to palliative care are reached by consensus, this method simply is not practical where a clinical management decision has to be made quickly, or when only one team member and the patient are involved, or in those unusual circumstances where agreement cannot be reached within the team. In health care in general many decisions are still based on the hierarchical model, and as a result the most senior member of the team is normally held accountable by professional organizations. A move towards more consensus decisions would logically entail more emphasis on the accountability of each individual, which would accord with an attitude of respect for the autonomy of all professionals.

From the legal point of view the most senior professional is usually held accountable for each aspect of care, following the hierarchical model described previously. For instance, the consultant is responsible for medical care in a hospital ward or palliative care unit, and the general practitioner has a parallel responsibility whilst the patient is at home. At the same time any individual doctor who falls short of professional standards may be reprimanded by his professional body and senior colleagues and in this sense is accountable for his or her decisions. The situation in nursing is more confused; there is a move to individual accountability in nursing and nurses do bear legal responsibility for their actions, but as yet nurses are rarely tried in court as individuals if their conduct is questioned. Instead, their employer is sued. This situation is logically likely to change as individual accountability is stressed by the profession itself. It is appropriate that all professionals play a part in decisions, but the greater the influence in the decision the greater is the degree of accountability for it. The price that nursing staff will have to pay for greater respect for their professional autonomy leading to a greater ability to influence decisions is a greater degree of accountability, and from the legal perspective this unfortunately means that they can and will be exposed to litigation.

An attitude of respect for the autonomy of each individual professional team member would entail a doctrine of absolute moral responsibility of each individual for his or her part in decision making and in delivering care. What then is the solution if there is a conflict of moral views within the team? Since individuals hold different values, and each has a unique background of professional experience, they may differ with regard to the management which they feel accords with the patient's medical good. They may also reach different conclusions in considering the balance of the patient's good versus that of the relative, or the balance between the interests of the patient and those of management, especially in terms of resource allocation. Other conflicts arise between the needs of the patient and the welfare of the team members and we shall discuss these later.

Various solutions to conflicts are possible, and there are several factors which are morally relevant in deciding which one is appropriate in a particular circumstance. If one disagrees with other members of the team, the first course of action is to listen carefully to the arguments on both sides, including the patient's point of view.

Respect for the autonomy of others demands that we recognize that they may have moral values which differ from our own, and therefore we respect their right to reach different conclusions in clinical decisions. It is obviously wrong to ridicule the considered opinions of professional colleagues or the patient. Once we have listened carefully to all the arguments, we should reconsider our own position, and we may have to modify our view accordingly. When working in a team we require open-mindedness, so that we listen to and hear the arguments of others.

Differences of view may occur between doctors in a patient-centred team. For example, an oncologist may consider that it is appropriate to give a jaundiced and very ill young man with a small cell carcinoma of the lung chemotherapy, on the basis that there is a very small chance of considerable benefit, and if the patient indicates he wants the treatment. However, the general practitioner and specialist in palliative medicine may consider that the young man is irreversibly dying and the chances of improvement are so small that any possible benefit is outweighed by the exhaustion and loss of valuable 'living time' entailed by repeated trips to the oncology department. Instead, they might consider that in this case chemotherapy should not have been offered. Ultimately the responsibility for giving this treatment lies with the oncologist, but it is important that the doctors concerned have the courage to talk together about their differences of opinion, since in the long run the patient's interests will best be served by sharing of the experience of the three doctors concerned.

Typical disagreements in palliative care surround the management of the incompetent patient, who may be confused or unconscious, where the responsibility for care rests entirely with the professional carers. Relatives can give valuable insights into the patient's values, but ultimately the responsibility for treatment decisions rests with the professionals who carry out the treatment. Conflict is particularly likely to occur between specialist palliative care nurses and general practitioners. This professional relationship is potentially fraught with problems because the nurse may be called upon to give advice about the control of symptoms, such as restlessness or pain, based on her considerable experience, but the ultimate responsibility for the treatment prescribed lies with the general practitioner, who has a background in pharmacology, and who has also probably known the patient and family for some years and has a greater insight into their values. On the other hand, the treatment prescribed by the doctor may be administered on some occasions by the nurse. In a case of conflict it is morally relevant who has the right and responsibility to make a decision.

If after discussion disagreement still persists and the doctor prescribes what the nurse feels to be an inadequate dose of analgesia, then she has no alternative but to accept this, and do what she can to make sure the patient is reviewed regularly so that the prescription can be changed. This is basically a damage-limitation strategy. It is applicable in situations where a decision has been made which has been a source of disagreement, usually because of uncertainty and moral complexity. Most clinical decisions have the potential to contribute to a bad outcome, especially in palliative care where the disease course is unpredictable and other circumstances change. What is important is that they are reviewed regularly and changed if the desired outcome is not being achieved.

Alternatively, if the doctor prescribes a combination of drugs which the nurse feels will cause overwhelming harm to the patient when balanced against possible benefit, and the nurse is instructed to implement this treatment, she has to decide whether to refuse. Before this drastic measure is taken she can tactfully suggest that advice from a specialist doctor may be helpful, or that another partner in the general practice might join in the discussion because the clinical situation is unusually difficult. If these measures fail, and she remains convinced that the prescription is harmful, she may refuse to give the medication. Indeed, she has a duty to challenge a prescription that she believes is manifestly wrong or unsafe. An alternative strategy is to give the medication and review the patient frequently— the damage-limitation approach. This is appropriate only if the drug is such that its full effect will occur gradually over a period of time rather than immediately, and that adverse effects are reversible if the treatment is withdrawn.

The scenario described above has arisen very occasionally where a doctor has prescribed large doses of sedatives and/or opiates and another professional colleague has believed that the intention was to shorten the patient's life. If that was the intention, then the prescribing doctor has acted illegally, and in a manner which is not morally condoned by the profession. In this particular circumstance it is right for the nurse to refuse to give the medication. Refusal to comply in this regard is an extreme position for a nurse to take, and her stance will probably cause the doctor to review his or her position. It is legally permissible for drugs to be used that will incidentally shorten life only if all the following three rules are obeyed:

1. the patient must already be dying,
2. the drugs must be 'right and proper' professional practice,
3. the motive must be to relieve pain, not shorten life.

In these situations of conflict the morally important aspects of the harms which may occur are the severity of the harm, the likelihood of the harm, and the extent to which it will be reversible or could be alleviated.

Other, less dramatic, situations arise where there is a moral conflict within the team about the balance of interests between the patient and relatives, for instance a spouse. This can occur if a patient wishes to be at home, where care can be provided by community services, but the spouse is called upon to perform non-skilled tasks such as giving drinks, doing the washing, and so on. Occasionally in this situation, particularly if the couple have not enjoyed a good relationship, the spouse may not want the patient to be at home, either because they do not get on well, or because the spouse is anxious, or perhaps does not want the patient to die at home and expresses fears about living in the house afterwards if this happens. If the patient is in hospital or a hospice, the team may be divided about whether the patient should be sent home against the wishes of the spouse.

No particular health care discipline has responsibility for this decision, which is essentially a team matter. Of course the easiest solution is for the couple to resolve it themselves, but there is a danger that a patient whose autonomy is compromised by ex-haustion and perhaps depression is overruled by a more autonomous spouse. The scenario of 'the survival of the most autonomous' may occur, whereby the interests of the most autonomous party override those of the least, even if the latter is the patient (see also Chapter 13, p. 278). There may be a majority team decision to endeavour to keep the patient in hospital, but some members may disagree and consider that the patient should be sent home (assuming that this is the patient's wish). Ultimately a decision must be reached, and this may be necessary before other circumstances intervene which could prevent discharge (such as a dramatic deterioration in medical condition). In this situation those who hold the minority view can voice their objections, and the fact that they are in the minority does not necessarily indicate that they are either wrong or right. The majority can also be right or wrong. Probably the minority should make a conscientious compromise and support the majority decision, although they should continue to try to limit the damage they perceive to the patient, perhaps by suggesting visits home or by encouraging the spouse to see the patient's point of view. For further discussion of this common problem see Chapter 3, p. 55.

It has been suggested that, where it is appropriate, nurses should adopt the role of 'patient's advocate'. This would mean that the nurse would always support the patient's point of view. But there are drawbacks to this policy. First, a nurse might be put in a position of having to advocate what she believed would harm the patient. Secondly, establishing an advocacy role for nurses would also divide the multidisciplinary team into nurses on one side (thought to be acting for the patient) and everyone else on the other (thought to be acting for other values). In fact, anyone close to the patient, whether professional or lay, could act as advocate. We do not consider that patient advocacy should be a role ascribed to nurses; such a policy would potentially deny the nurse her own professional autonomy, and would create practical as well as ideological divisions between professionals.

Where major conflict occurs between one team member and the rest, and a conscientious compromise is not possible, that member may feel sufficiently strongly to resign. Occasionally a professional may feel that the philosophy and conduct of the team to which they belong is so much at variance with the demands of their own conscience that resignation is the only appropriate course. From the professional's point of view resignation has the advantage of ensuring removal from the moral conflict situation. The disadvantage is that if the professional considers that patients are being harmed by the conduct of the team then resignation will do nothing to further their cause. The alternative of remaining in the team and trying to change the views of colleagues so as to improve patient care should be considered, although the personal costs could be high.

Rarely, professionals have resigned in circumstances where they feel that management, in an attempt to reduce costs, has compromised the quality of patient care to an unacceptable degree. Whilst this extreme step does register a protest, it carries the disadvantage of removing one dissenting voice from the discussion which is then more likely to be overwhelmed by the management initiative. It is probably preferable in terms of consequences for the patients to remain in one's post and to strive continually for the patients' good, but again the personal costs will be high.

Standing up for one's own personal values or perhaps those of one's profession requires moral courage. This is especially true if one is in a minority position, if the decision which others have chosen is effectively an 'easier way out', or if voicing one's criticisms could result in adverse career consequences because those with whom one disagrees are in a position of power and will be called upon to provide future references. The moral quality of courage is required. This quality is of great value in health care; those who do stand up for their own views stimulate discussion which is most likely to lead to the best results for patient care, and sometimes it is only the courage of a single professional which saves a patient from harm at the hands of other misguided colleagues.

4.7 Moral deficiency

Serious professional misdemeanours are disciplinary offences, and may also constitute a breach of the law. In palliative care such occurrences are fortunately very rare, and they will not be considered further here, except to say that they should be reported because our duty first and foremost is to patient welfare.

Much more commonly a professional colleague falls short of the high standards of palliative care by exhibiting an inappropriate attitude to the patient or to other colleagues. They may show a lack of compassion or honesty, or be arrogant or patronizing. They may be quick to anger or rude, or they may simply stir up trouble surreptitiously in the team or be prone to spread unkind gossip. In the close-knit nuclear model of the team this behaviour is likely to be noticed and commented on by other individuals, but to do this is not enough—a solution to the problem should be sought.

It may be necessary for the team to acknowledge the difficulty openly and try to resolve it by discussion with the person concerned. Alternatively it may be appropriate to notify the carer's senior colleague confidentially. In both cases any reason for the undesirable attitude and behaviour should be sought. Moral failures may be due to emotional exhaustion or depression, which may be exacerbated by overwhelming difficulties in the personal life of the carer. In this case understanding is required plus whatever practical assistance can be given to help, including sick leave if appropriate. If the inappropriate attitude is intrinsic to the personality of the carer, the problem may be very difficult to resolve. Explanation and argument about adverse consequences of the attitude for patients and colleagues may help and should be tried. If they prove ineffective and the person concerned is destructive to the team and to patient welfare, they should be dismissed if possible, but if regulations preclude this, then movement to a position of lesser influence is required. This constitutes a damage-limitation strategy.

4.8   Caring for each other

Respecting the autonomy of our colleagues entails 'making their ends our own'. This means having regard to their vision of their welfare as we do our own. If we have this attitude we will show concern and give what practical help we can to our colleagues when they need it. Usually we do not need to consider this duty when a fellow team member is distressed—our desire to help springs from the affection and regard we have developed for them over time. It may be necessary to remind ourselves of the attitude of respect for autonomy when our natural desire to help is lessened by previous friction or disagreements or perhaps personal dislike.

Palliative care is emotionally stressful for all staff, and can also be physically very demanding for nursing staff. We have a duty to support each other, and if an individual is particularly vulnerable due to temporary personal circumstances or recent distressing incidents at work, then colleagues should take some steps to lighten his or her load for a while. Good advice for those who are temporarily undergoing increased stress is 'do not walk the extra mile with patients or colleagues'.

On the other hand, if a fellow team member is unable to sustain his or her workload over a long period, or manages to do so but only at the cost of continuing physical exhaustion or mental distress, then a more difficult moral problem exists. Even if patient care does not suffer, the carer is obviously being harmed. Unfortunately, this may be obvious to the rest of the team but not to the individual who is suffering. A misguided idea of loyalty or kindness may prevent other team members from drawing attention to the problem with the individual and with management. Emotional exhaustion or 'burn out' is not uncommon in those involved in palliative care. It may be due to a strong motivation to do one's best for the patient no matter what the personal cost, or to frustration at not being able to do the job as well as one would like, usually due to resource constraints. Unrealistic goals, which may be inappropriate anyway (such as wanting angry, struggling people to die calmly and reconciled to their death as well as their life) may also contribute.

Whilst we all want the best for our patients, specialist palliative care for professionals is not about martyrdom. Most of us do not feel called to a life of complete dedication to patient care. There are some saintly persons who are able to devote their entire lives to those terminally ill and still remain well-balanced and fully developed people, but they are few. For ordinary mortals, rest and relaxation and a normal home-life away from the job are essential for mental health and development. For most of us, total and exclusive dedication to palliative care will result in emotional exhaustion and perhaps longer term damage. Such martyrdom will not help in the long term, because experienced, effective, and compassionate carers may have to leave specialist work as a result of emotional exhaustion. Moreover, we know that we will need specialists in this important area for the foreseeable future; if the first generation of doctors and nurses to undertake palliative care as a lifetime career show an alarming tendency to succumb to 'burn out', then the next generation may not come forward to follow on.

If a fellow team member is obviously in difficulties, others need to approach him or her tactfully to offer to understand and to help. If it is thought that such offers may be rebuffed, then a senior colleague and/or manager of the person in difficulties should be informed about the perceived problem. Where the person concerned is a consultant or nurse manager in an independent hospice, there may seem to be nowhere to turn for help, except perhaps to other senior members of the team with whom the person enjoys a good relationship. Within the National Health Service there are procedures for dealing with such problems, and personnel departments should be used for the valuable help they can provide.

If a carer is unable to sustain the professional task, patient care will ultimately suffer, but the other equally important moral reason for assisting a distressed team member is that, as St Paul says, we are members one of another.

4.9 Conclusions

1. A patient-centred concept of teamwork is practically and morally preferable to the managerial concept of a tightly bonded and bounded group.

2. There are various senses in which team members can be held responsible for their actions, and in which the team as a whole may be collectively responsible for its actions.

3. When conflict persists in the team after open-minded discussion, a consensus decision can be reached only by conscientious compromises on behalf of some members.

4. Rarely, it may be appropriate for a professional to refuse to implement a decision which he or she strongly feels is morally wrong on the grounds that it is likely to cause serious and irreversible harm.

5. Inappropriate attitudes and behaviour of professional team members should be discussed with the person concerned, and attempts made to alter them by explanation and argument. If this fails, the team member should be moved or encouraged to leave because ultimately the quality of patient care is paramount.

6. We have a duty of care to professional colleagues; this arises from respect for their autonomy, and from the kind of love called *agape*.

5

Process of clinical decision making

Read not to contradict and confute, nor to believe and take for granted, nor to find talk and discourse, but to weigh and consider.

Francis Bacon, *Essays*, 'Of Studies' (1625)

What is a 'good' clinical decision? For practising clinicians, the question 'How can I make better decisions?' is seen to be highly relevant, and crucial to our aim of being a better doctor, nurse, or other professional. We need to establish the moral criteria by which a decision is judged, that is, what is 'better' about a good decision than a bad one.

In previous chapters we have stressed that the desired *outcome* of our care is the patient's total good, or best interests, which comprises their medical good interpreted in the light of their own goals and values. If the patient's wishes cannot be known because the patient is not autonomous or is unable to communicate, and has left no advance directive or proxy, then we act in accordance with the patient's medical good, balancing the risks and burdens of treatment against the benefits. This chapter begins by examining our responsibility for outcomes and then deals mainly with the *process* of decision making. We shall endeavour to clarify the moral issues which arise in the traditional methods of decision making, and explore the moral difficulties inherent in the use of some more recently developed formal systems such as flow charts and clinical guidelines which have been proposed as improvements on the traditional process. In palliative care we have to make decisions in circumstances which entail factual complexities, uncertainties, and difficult moral choices. Nevertheless, a decision has to be made. We may make a conscious decision to postpone making a particular choice—for instance, we often postpone a decision until the disease course becomes more obvious—but we cannot avoid making any decision at all.

5.1 Responsibility and outcome

It is often said that we are 'morally responsible' for our decisions. What does it mean to be 'morally responsible' for a clinical decision? It is important to understand the various senses of the word 'responsible', all of which relate to the morality of decision making.

In the first sense we speak of one person being *responsible to* another person or group; as doctors we are responsible to our managers for the way our drug budget is used, and a ward nurse is responsible to the ward sister for the care of her patients. This means that the doctor or nurse is accountable to the manager and ward sister respectively, in the sense that they are obliged to explain and justify their actions.

In the second sense we speak of a person being *responsible for* something. The doctor is responsible for the way the drug budget is spent, and the nurse is responsible for the care of her patients. This use of the word does not necessarily entail being accountable to someone. For instance, the doctor and nurse are both personally responsible for their own health. What a person is responsible for in this sense may be called *responsibilities*. The clinical medical and nursing care of patients is often referred to as the responsibility of the doctor and nurse respectively.

Sometimes we use the word in a third sense as an adjective. We may say that a junior nurse or doctor is responsible, meaning that he or she is reliable and conscientious, or *has a sense of responsibility*.

In a fourth sense, a person may be *causally responsible* for an event. For instance, if a nurse slips on the floor and accidentally knocks a patient over she would be causally responsible for the patient falling down, but she would not be held 'morally' responsible or blameworthy for it. If, on the other hand, she caused the patient to fall by deliberately failing to support the patient during lifting, then she would definitely be considered both causally and morally responsible for the fall.

Finally, we may say that a person's responsibility was impaired, meaning that he was not capable of making up making up his own mind about what he ought or ought not to do. In other words, he was not autonomous. In all the other senses, except simply causing something to happen, it is assumed that a person is already responsible in this sense, or is autonomous. *To be autonomous is*

to be individually responsible or accountable for one's behaviour.
We assume that, unless mentally ill or being coerced in some way,
professional carers are responsible or autonomous in their decisions.
We tend to use the word 'responsible' in all these ways when
discussing clinical decisions, and its multiple uses are a source of
potential confusion, as we shall now show.

Since the progress of a disease is unpredictable, and many factors
other than our treatment bring about outcomes such as the patient's
death or distress, we may or may not be causally responsible for everything that happens after a clinical decision, that is for the *outcome*.
This is so because the care we gave following a decision either to
do something or not to do it is only one factor in the outcome.
Outcomes in palliative care are the result of many factors acting
together. Our action (or inaction, if we decided not to do something)
is therefore often only a partial cause of the overall outcome. Therefore, we are often only partially responsible in the simple causal
sense for the outcome, and we cannot then be held entirely morally
responsible for the outcome. This is what we mean when we say
someone was only partially *morally responsible* for an outcome.

In the context of palliative care, lack of understanding of the
meaning of the term 'responsible for' in different contexts has caused
considerable confusion which has unfortunately led to incorrect
conclusions about causal responsibility and blameworthiness. For
instance, a doctor may have chosen not to give a frail and terminally
ill patient antibiotics. The doctor is responsible for this decision in
the sense that the decision was made as a result of clinical judgement.
However, if the patient dies, that death is the result of a combination
of factors, such as a debilitated condition making overwhelming
infection more likely to occur and likely to be fatal, and the terminal
nature of the illness itself. It cannot be known if giving antibiotics
would have made any difference to the outcome of the pneumonia,
although doing so might have helped to overcome this infection and
so prolong life. The doctor is causally responsible for the patient's
death only to the extent that not giving antibiotics contributed to
the death. Therefore, whilst the doctor is fully responsible for the
decision, he or she is only partly causally responsible for the outcome, and so can be only partly responsible in a blameworthy or
praiseworthy sense for the patient's death.

This is a controversial position, because some parties have
maintained that if a treatment such as antibiotics is omitted in this

situation, then the doctor is directly and entirely causally responsible for the patient's death, and is either blameworthy or praiseworthy (according to your point of view) on that account. But on the basis of our professional knowledge of palliative care we would consider that this death, like most deaths, was multifactorial in origin. The doctor was causal in only one factor, that is the absence of antibiotics, and it is not even certain that this omission influenced the outcome at all, since the patient may well have succumbed even with antibiotics because of the very great influence of factors related to advanced terminal disease. It is on these grounds that we reject the argument that omitting a treatment which could perhaps prolong life *necessarily* makes the doctor causally responsible for the patients death and therefore either blameworthy or praiseworthy on account of that death. For a more detailed discussion of this topic refer to Chapter 13, p. 270.

In palliative care it is very important to be aware of the distinctions between:

1. being entirely causally responsible for an outcome, in the sense that one's action or inaction directly and of itself caused the outcome to happen;
2. being partly causally responsible for that outcome which in fact resulted from the interaction of many factors one of which was one's action or inaction;
3. being either blameworthy or praiseworthy on account of the outcome, which is logically possible only if one's action or inaction was to some extent the cause of the outcome. Obviously, the extent to which one may be blameworthy or praiseworthy for the outcome depends on the extent to which one's action or inaction directly contributed to the outcome.

In palliative care we are only occasionally entirely causally responsible for an outcome, and therefore fully morally responsible for that outcome. Usually, we are only partly causally responsible for the outcome, and can therefore be only partly morally responsible in the sense of attribution of blame or praise on account of the outcome. In contrast, we are entirely responsible for the *process* by which we make the decision, and are rightly held to be accountable for the factors we consider and the way in which we balance their importance.

In law, however, one may be treated as wholly blameworthy or praiseworthy even when only partially causally responsible. An inaction may also be culpable if death may result.

Those professionals involved in palliative care are only too aware of the extent of uncertainty with regard to the influence that our interventions actually have over the outcome. We simply do not know whether many of the things we do make a difference or not. This is one of the reasons why it is misleading to pass a moral judgement on our decision *solely* on the basis of the outcome. For the remainder of the chapter we shall concentrate on the process of decision making. This is the location of our main moral responsibility, although, as we shall see, there are constraints even here.

5.2   Responsibility and process

The process of reaching a clinical decision has two stages; the first involves understanding the clinical problem, and the second involves using our reason to work out the best solution in the light of various constraints on clinical freedom, and in the hope of finding a consensus.

5.2.1   *Understanding the problem*

This involves knowing what information is relevant, gathering that information, and assimilating it or 'taking it on board' so that it can be carefully considered. Sometimes we fail to make a good decision because we do not appreciate that some information is relevant, and therefore either fail to obtain it, fail to believe it, or fail to use it in the decision. A great deal of knowledge is of importance in even apparently simple decisions.

Scientific factual knowledge is required. This includes knowledge of the diagnosis, or failing that of the apparent symptoms and signs, as well as the natural history, of the illness. Similar knowledge of the available treatments and their associated benefits, risks, and burdens is part of our basic professional expertise. This sort of knowledge has the generality of all scientific knowledge. We then require some knowledge about the patient's social background such as occupational and family history, and present social circumstances. This kind of social science based knowledge gives us understanding in the sense that we can fit the patient's profile into a pattern which tells us how similar patients with similar illnesses have been affected and have reacted.

But whilst we have said that the *science* of palliative care is about similarities, the *art* of such care lies in addressing the particularities or uniqueness of each patient's situation. We therefore need information and understanding about this particular situation, relating both to this illness and this patient. This information is individualized. A certain amount of such knowledge is derived from the case history, which is about how the illness developed and progressed in this patient. Finally, as the last component of our understanding, we need imaginative and intuitive insight into the meaning of this illness for this person, as described in Chapter 1. This includes trying to ascertain the outcomes that the patient seeks, together with his or her own opinion of their priorities.

Where the patient is largely non-autonomous, as a result of confusion or because information has been declined or denied, or where the patient has no autonomy as when unconscious or totally confused perhaps due to a cerebral tumour or advanced dementia, then the carer still requires all the scientific understanding of the problems, and should seek some individualized understanding from relatives and friends of the patient as to the patient's story, together with some idea of what his or her wishes might have been.

The practical difficulties of doing this are well-known to those who have tried. Relatives often find it very hard to say 'what the patient would have wanted', or are reluctant to take partial responsibility for the decision by so doing. A statement about what the patient would have wanted is called a substitute judgement, and some relatives find it a difficult concept to grasp. They may want to recommend only that treatment which they think is in the patient's interests, or may quite naturally be influenced by their own personal interests. Nonetheless some attempt should be made to ascertain what the patient might have wanted in the situation, and information gained should influence the ultimate decision in the direction of their overall well-being. In other words, as much understanding of the patient's situation as possible should be gained.

In addition, where the patient is not autonomous and family and friends bear the burden of caring, then their interests also become relevant. Understanding of the patient's problems is then not complete without some appreciation of the needs of those on whom they are dependent. For example, a confused or demented patient who is also physically very frail is often dependent entirely on his or her spouse plus visiting professionals for care. If the spouse is simply not willing or able to undertake the demands of such care, then this must strongly influence decisions on further management. This situation is common and very difficult to resolve. The patient is totally vulnerable, and there is a risk that whoever has autonomy will get their wishes respected at the expense of the patient's total good. The professional's task is to strive for the patient's good, influenced by anything that might be known of the patient's values, but the willingness and ability of the family to shoulder the burden of care is a necessary constraint in making the decision and so needs to be known and accepted.

The following example illustrates the elements which comprise understanding the particular problem. A specialist in palliative medicine was asked to visit an elderly man urgently at home. His condition seemed to have deteriorated rapidly. He was known to have extensive bone metastases from carcinoma of the prostate gland, but he also suffered from severe Parkinson's disease for which he had been on regular oral medication. When seen he was unable to speak and was completely rigid and immobile—a couple of days earlier he had become unable to take his oral medication for Parkinson's disease, due to nausea and general deterioration in his condition, and as a result he had become completely immobile and unable to communicate. Prior to this his condition had been deteriorating with markedly increasing weakness and profound anorexia. There was no way to administer oral medications for his Parkinson's disease at home and his wife and the community nurses were having difficulty meeting his care needs, partly due to his extreme immobility. It proved impossible to ascertain his wishes as he was unable to communicate.

Scientific understanding of the problem related to knowledge of the natural history of prostate cancer and Parkinson's disease, and the treatments available for both conditions. In particular, it was important to know that all treatments for Parkinson's disease are oral medications apart from apomorphine given subcutaneously, which requires specialist advice. Understanding of his particular situation also required knowledge about the progress of the illnesses in his case. It was relevant that from the history of his illness he seemed to be in the process of dying from his carcinomatosis.

The patient's social circumstances were also relevant—his wife was devoted and his five sons, some of whom had not seen him recently, were scattered around the world. His wife was willing to continue to care for him at home if this was considered the best option for him. The question arose as to whether he should be nursed as well as possible at home, without oral or artificial hydration, and with whatever medications were necessary for his comfort administered subcutaneously. It was considered too hazardous to try to pass a nasogastric tube at home because of his swallowing difficulties due to his Parkinson's disease. The alternative was to admit him to a specialist palliative care unit and there to pass a nasogastric tube to administer medications for his Parkinson's disease or to use apomorphine with specialist advice. The option of artificial hydration was also available in such a unit.

His wife was asked to say what she thought his wishes might be in the circumstances. In other words, she was asked to try to make a substitute judgement. Initially, she found this impossible. Consequently, she was asked if she could describe his general approach to life and characteristic attitudes. She said that he had always been 'a fighter', a statement which suggested that more active treatment in the palliative care unit with possible prolongation of life might have been his wish. However, when asked what he fought for, she said he had always been independent and active despite his illnesses and that he disliked and dreaded dependency. Therefore, she considered that he might not have wanted his life prolonged in what was inevitably going to be a dependent condition. When asked about his attitude to family relationships she said he had always been close to his sons, and was very much a 'family man'. She felt he might want the opportunity to see them again, and on further consideration she decided that this would probably have been his priority in the circumstances, even if it entailed having life prolonged in a dependent condition.

In the United Kingdom the responsibility for making decisions for incompetent patients lies with the health care team. After consideration of all the above relevant aspects of the problem, they decided to admit the patient to a specialist palliative care unit, where a nasogastric tube was passed (with some difficulty) by an anaesthetist, and medication for his Parkinson's disease and some fluid were administered. His condition improved a little, so that he was able to speak and move with assistance in bed, and his sons returned from around the world. Fortunately he was able to talk with them for a few days before his condition deteriorated again and he died.

This clinical example illustrates the process of deciding what treatment options might further the patient's medical good, and then considering what his own goals and values in the particular situation might have been. The latter is often a very difficult judgement to form. Finally, a decision about his total good is made by consideration of medical good combined with what can reasonably be surmised about what his wishes might have been.

The task of the health care team after understanding the patient's problem is to select treatment options and then reach a consensus, involving the patient whenever possible, as to which is the best in the circumstances. However, there are constraints on the professional's clinical freedom when selecting treatment options and it is important to consider these.

5.2.2 *Clinical freedom*

As professionals our ability to act in what we believe to be the patient's best interests is sometimes referred to as clinical freedom. We all know that clinical freedom exists only within the bounds of certain *constraints*. First, there are those of human and financial resources, and some necessary managerial constraints, such as how staff are deployed. We shall discuss this further in Chapters 9 and 12.

A second necessary constraint on clinical freedom is the moral requirement to act justly. Some aspects of this principle are enshrined by our community in laws, and obviously our decisions must result in acts within the law. In palliative care the most relevant legal constraints are the laws surrounding informed consent and the prohibition against (intentional) killing. The law in both cases is based on the interests of society as a whole, as well as on the interests of individual patients.

A third constraint on clinical freedom derives from the purchaser–provider system of health care. This constraint is found when the purchaser of care imposes conditions relating to clinical practice, such as treatment protocols or clinical guidelines, on the professional providers of care via the contract. Contracts between purchasers and independent providers of care such as charitably funded hospices are legal documents and as such are legally binding. Contracts between NHS hospital trusts as providers and purchasers are also enforceable, though only through arbitration, not through the courts. It is likely that in trying to ensure the most cost-effective care, the purchasers may insist via the contract that certain treatment protocols are followed. It is obvious that this greatly reduces the available options of treatment for the patient. Treatment according to the protocol may be entirely inappropriate for a particular patient. This scenario is unfortunately very likely to occur in palliative care, where individual requirements vary. Moreover, terminally ill patients have by definition little time left to live; if one treatment given according to the protocol fails, there will probably not be time to try another. Therefore, adherence to the protocol may deny patient and carer the only opportunity they have to make decisions in accordance with the patient's total good, which is the aim of palliative care.

The art of decision making in palliative care lies in the choice of treatment for a particular patient, whereas protocols and clinical guidelines are about the generality of patients, and whilst they inform the decision by stating knowledge derived from statistics, they cannot alone dictate the appropriate treatment or care plan for a particular patient.

Furthermore, since it seems uncertain whether the purchaser bears moral or legal responsibility for the treatment given to a particular patient, it is difficult to see how imposition of certain treatments or care plans is either morally or legally justifiable. The purchaser will not be considered blameworthy or be sued because inappropriate care was given. We make this point strongly because we believe that imposition of certain treatments or care plans by purchasers threatens the whole ethos of palliative care; it prevents the carer from acting from an attitude of beneficence, and it shows no respect for either carer's or patient's autonomy. It seems that this fact has been little recognized and its importance will not be appreciated until dire consequences for particular patients have ensued.

A fourth constraint on clinical freedom arises when the patient is no longer able to make his or her own decisions due to diminished consciousness or confusion, or is totally unable to communicate, as with very severe dysphasia. In such cases the relatives may feel that they know best what is in the patient's interests and/or what the patient would have wanted. The relatives may also state their own interests in decisions regarding the patient. It is sometimes very difficult for those close to the patient to distinguish between these three influences, which interact and together result in the relatives' opinions as to what should be done. It must be understood that legally in the United Kingdom a relative or next of kin cannot consent to treatment on behalf of the adult patient. In other countries the law may give relatives varying degrees of decision-making authority for incompetent patients. The extent to which the wishes of relatives should be taken into account in clinical decisions is much debated and is a source of great confusion. This topic is discussed in Chapter 3, p. 58.

Unfortunately, since litigation has increased in most areas of health care, and the fear of it has increased even more, it is easy for professionals to be strongly influenced by what the relatives feel is in the patient's best interests. This is especially so in palliative care where the patient is often not in a position to act as a witness. This concern may encourage such treatments as intravenous or sub-cutaneous hydration for an unconscious dying patient where the professional opinion is that such treatment would not be advantageous physiologically, might actually be harmful if renal or cardiac failure is likely, and is very unlikely to increase patient comfort. The fear of litigation can unfortunately give the relatives' opinion in this case more weight in the decision than it should have, and professionals may feel coerced by the (usually unstated) threat of litigation into doing what they feel is either futile or actually harmful to the patient. Fortunately, overt threats of litigation by relatives are rare in palliative care, but fear of litigation is a constraint, and may on occasion lead to inappropriate treatment.

Similar difficulties may arise if relatives wish to influence care in the direction of their own best interests. This is legitimate if they are directly involved in the practical care of the patient, in which case they are free to choose what they may or may not undertake. On the other hand, it is arguable to what extent they should influence professional care for their own financial interests. For example, it may uncommonly happen that a relative has a vested financial interest in the date a patient dies, perhaps because of an insurance policy. They may then want to influence treatment decisions which could prolong life. We think that in this situation the professional carers should act in accordance with the patient's best interests; such a rule is necessary to protect vulnerable patients from harm which would occur to them if relatives were given sway over life-prolonging treatment in this situation.

A fifth constraint on clinical freedom can arise where the patient's care has to be funded out of his or her own assets which means that future beneficiaries of the estate stand to lose financially. Recently in the United Kingdom patients who need a protected environment and/or nursing care have to fund this out of their own resources if they can afford to do so. Relatives who may stand to inherit much-needed funds from the patient obviously have a vested interest in the patient not going into residential care. Whilst in the United Kingdom it is government policy that terminally ill patients thought to be close to death are entitled to a hospital bed, shortage of these beds forces professional carers to suggest that stable patients whose needs could be met in retirement homes or nursing homes should go there so as to liberate hospital beds for those whose needs cannot otherwise be met. Therefore, terminally ill patients are transferred to nursing homes. In this very difficult situation professional carers may feel coerced by relatives not to institute or continue life-prolonging treatment which would increase the nursing home bills.

Fortunately, this problem again is rare in practice because life-prolonging treatment is often futile in terminally ill patients, and is in addition often very burdensome to confused patients, and so it is not in accord with the patient's medical good. Where it does arise, professionals may feel very reluctant to prolong the patient's life if the costs of so doing are going to be seriously detrimental to relatives, particularly the elderly spouse of the patient who may have a very low income. This sort of pressure on the carer does amount to a constraint on clinical freedom.

5.2.3   Reaching solutions

Within the constraints just discussed the professional task of decision making requires the carer to select treatment options which accord with the patient's medical good in order to offer those options to the patient. This selection is made on the basis of understanding of the particular situation, and on professional knowledge and experience. Care options might include various methods of symptom control plus solutions to practical problems of care, and perhaps advice about approaches to social, psychological, or spiritual problems if the patient has requested help with such difficulties.

Should carers offer treatment which they do not feel would contribute to this patient's medical good but which is generally available? This question has arisen partly in response to public demand for more control and choice in care, and partly because of legal documents like the Patient's Charter which stress that patients have a right to be told of *all* treatments available for their condition, plus the risks, burdens, and benefits of those treatments. This issue is now highly contentious.

We think that the requirement in the Patient's Charter that patients should be told of all the treatment options and their risks and benefits should be interpreted as applying to each case individually. In other words the carer's professional duty is to suggest those options which accord with this particular patient's medical good, as a basis for discussion.

Since the professional is held accountable for giving the treatment, then he or she must have a choice as to whether to offer and give it or not. In other words, the carer must have complete clinical freedom in this kind of decision. If the professional must ultimately do whatever the patient asks, as in the customer–salesperson relationship model (pp. 8, 41, and 279), then the professional cannot be held accountable for giving the treatment and for its consequences. If professional clinical freedom is to be respected, then carers must be able to refuse to give treatment which they believe would cause more harm than good, that is where the burdens and/or risks greatly outweigh the benefits. For example, surgeons must be permitted to refuse to perform operations, such as oesophagectomy or lung lobectomy to resect tumours, if they believe that the benefits of surgery in the particular case are outweighed by its harms and risks.

In summary, assessment of medical good by the professional entails a benefits to burdens/risks calculus based on relevant knowledge as described above. The professional should offer treatment options which:

1. offer good or reasonable hope of benefit with low or moderate burdens or risks which are explained to the patient;
2. offer good or reasonable hope of benefit with high burdens or risks, which are explained to the patient, and advice is given;
3. offer minimal likelihood of benefit with low or moderate burdens or risks which are explained to the patient. If the professional feels that in their opinion burdens and risks may outweigh the benefit, they have a duty as professionals to advise the patient of this;

4. offer a small chance of a major benefit, such as cure, much improved
   quality of life, or significant prolongation of life, even if associated burdens and risks are great, since some people would wish to
   accept great burdens and risks for a small chance of a major benefit.

The professional should *not* offer care options which may have a
minimal benefit in some cases but which they feel *in this case* would
entail overwhelming burdens/risks in comparison to the very small
chance of benefit. Treatments should not be offered if the professional feels they would be physiologically ineffective, even if they are
sometimes used in the illness. For example, radiotherapy where a
tumour has already shown radioresistance should not be offered. There
is no obligation to offer treatment which is futile in this respect.

In addition, it does not seem reasonable for the professional to be
bound to offer treatments which he or she would not be prepared to
give on the grounds of overwhelming burdens or risks in comparison
with only some chance of a *minor* benefit. In contrast, as stated
above, treatments with a small chance of a *major* benefit should be
offered, with explanation about burdens and risks and some advice
about the unique situation under discussion.

For instance, where there is a form of chemotherapy which carries
a small possibility of disease response (giving prolongation of life for
some months—not cure), but a very high possibility of severe side-
effects such as malaise and nausea, together with a significant risk of
life-threatening infection following marrow depression, it does not
seem reasonable to maintain that the professional should offer such
treatment. There are two reasons for this; firstly, the benefits to
burdens/risk calculus in this case concludes that there is a very great
chance of harm, and very little chance of benefit, and thus the
treatment would not seem to be in accord with the patient's medical
good, and secondly because on these grounds the professional would
be unwilling to administer it. It seems illogical to offer treatment for
which the benefits to burdens/risks calculus so overwhelmingly
indicates an outcome of harm that the professional would not and
should not be willing to carry it out.

It is evident that in offering advice the professional requires the
moral quality of practical wisdom, discussed in Chapter 1. Since
giving such advice for which one is held accountable is the essence of
being a professional, *phronesis* or practical wisdom is the quality to
which we should aspire. Such practical wisdom enables the carer to

| QUANTITY | | | | TERMS | | SHIP VIA | |
| SHIPPED | BACKORDER | ISBN | TITLE/AUTHOR/EDITION | PRICE | DISCOUNT | NET AMOUNT | |

QUANTITY			TERMS NET 30 DAYS			SHIP VIA UPS	
SHIPPED	BACKORDER	ISBN	TITLE/AUTHOR/EDITION	PRICE	DISCOUNT	NET AMOUNT	
1	0	0-7876-2947-2	GREAT AMERICAN COURT CASES 4V HUBBARD 01	350.00	5.0	332.50	
1	0	0-7876-2948-0	GREAT AMERICAN COURT CASES V1 HUBBARD 01	.00		.00.	
1	0	0-7876-2949-9	GREAT AMERICAN COURT CASES V2 HUBBARD 01	.00		.00	
1	0	0-7876-2950-2	GREAT AMERICAN COURT CASES V3 HUBBARD 01	.00		.00	
1	0	0-7876-2951-0	GREAT AMERICAN COURT CASES V4 HUBBARD 01	.00		.00	
4	BOOKS						

120399

01/26/00   NET 30 DAYS

RECEIVED

SUBTOTAL	332.50
MISC. CHARGES	.00
SALES TAX	.00
SHIP & HANDLING	16.64

RETURNS POLICY

PLEASE SEND RETURNS TO THE "RETURN BOOKS TO" ADDRESS BELOW [YOU WILL BE
CHARGED FOR HANDLING RETURNS SENT TO AN INCORRECT ADDRESS]. SHIP ONLY UNUSED

Donna Page

see the good in the particular situation. Other moral qualities such as courage, integrity, and compassion also help us the see the right course, and then to carry it out.

5.2.4   *Reaching a consensus*

Where the patient is largely *autonomous* there is usually no difficulty in reaching a consensus decision between patient and carer about the right course of action. On rare occasions continuing disagreement occurs, and in this situation the autonomy of both parties is respected in that the patient cannot have treatment imposed if he or she does not want it, and the professional cannot be forced to give treatment which he or she feels is not in accord with the patient's medical good.

Some difficulties may also arise with regard to the interest of relatives which may conflict with those of the patient. In other words, pursuit of the patient's total good may not accord with the good of relatives.

This is a particular problem in palliative care where the philosophy of care often stated regards the entire family as the unit of care. This view inevitably means that conflicts of interest between patient and relatives become almost unresolvable, because each is given equal priority. We believe that the patient's total good must have priority in the mind of the carer because this aim is intrinsic to being a carer. This does not mean that relatives' views and interests should not be taken into account by both patient and carer. For further discussion of this problem, see Chapter 3.

The relatives' interests, however, do become a legitimate consideration and justifiably must strongly influence the decision where the patient is physically dependent on them for care. In this situation the relatives must be asked what care they feel they are willing and able to undertake, and a management plan cannot be suggested if the relatives feel unwilling and/or unable to shoulder the burden of care it entails. It must be stressed that if the patient is being expected to make decisions about care, then he or she must be informed of the relevant facts which include the ability of relatives to undertake both practical and emotional aspects of care. Ideally, such a discussion should be a family affair.

Sometimes relatives feel unable and/or unwilling to undertake the burdens of care but are reluctant to say this to the patient. They may then ask professionals to invent or exaggerate a medical reason for going into residential care, either hospital, specialist palliative care unit, or nursing home. But anything less than honesty in this situation is contrary to respect for the patient's autonomy. The philosophy of palliative care has always stressed the importance of the patient's dignity: maintaining dignity in this situation entails giving the patient the necessary information to make his or her own decision. We should not be dishonest with the patient in order to make a difficult choice easier for the relatives.

If the patient is judged incompetent in respect of a decision, then the professional task is once again to judge what is in the patient's best interests or total good, taking into consideration the patient's medical good and his or her own wishes. They may ask the relatives to give some indication of what the patient's wishes might have been. If the relatives feel unable to do this, or do not want to take the responsibility of influencing the decision by doing so, then some indication of the patient's values and priorities helps professionals to choose treatment which might accord with the patient's total good.

Instructions given via advance directives (living wills) should be respected if it is thought that the circumstances which have arisen are those the patient envisaged when the directive was written, and if, so far as can be ascertained, the patient was informed and competent to make such a choice when the directive was written. Advance directives will be discussed in detail later (pp. 191–96).

5.3 Three logical distinctions in decision making

Our discussion of the process of decision making has involved the factors involved in understanding the patient's problem, and in reaching solutions or at least in deciding treatment options. We shall now outline three ethical, or perhaps logical, distinctions which are often employed in the process of decision making in palliative care: the distinctions between intended and foreseen consequences, acts and omissions, and killing and letting die.

5.3.1 *Intended and foreseen consequences: doctrine of double effect*

In palliative care we have stressed that the carer's intention must be to cause overall benefit which contributes to the patient's total good, and we have stressed that treatment options should be offered following a benefits to burdens/risks calculus. Burdens and risks are foreseen but not intended. Since one is accountable for one's advice and for treatment given, foreseen burdens and risks entailed in the treatment proposed must be justified by the relative benefit. This is so with virtually all medical and nursing interventions.

In situations of severe distress such as mental anguish, restlessness, or unrelieved pain, autonomous patients may ask for or be offered sedation. This is given with the intention of alleviating distress; the sedation achieves this aim by decreasing mental anguish or lessening the patient's awareness of it. The autonomous patient can make such a decision with the caring team. Sedation is usually intermittent, allowing times of greater alertness to enjoy company, fluid and food, and facilitating changes of position. However, if distress is so severe as to require greater sedation if it is to be relieved, then there is a significant risk that life may be shortened. Nevertheless, the caring team may still offer the treatment and the patient may accept it following the benefits to burdens/risks calculus in this case. The benefit of alleviating severe distress is considered by patients and carers to outweigh the possible harm of shortening the duration of the terminal illness. Sedation sufficient to alleviate distress is used. Intentional overdoses of either analgesics or sedative medication are not morally justified.

Non-autonomous patients who are confused or paranoid may be given antipsychotic drugs to alleviate their agitation, and this sometimes cannot be achieved without drowsiness as an additional effect. Occasionally, in the case of patients with cerebral tumours, severe fitting may also necessitate continuous infusion of midazolam which causes sedation. Frequently, alertness diminishes at the end of life and agitation and restlessness with some confusion ensue. In all of these cases the caring team must again weigh the benefits of alleviating the patient's distress against the risks of shortening life. It is generally accepted that in those who are terminally ill the great benefits of alleviating such suffering by sedation, if all else has failed, outweigh the harm entailed in the risk of shortening life. This is a straightforward application of the benefits to burdens/risks calculus in decision making.

However, society prohibits its members from intentional killing and acts which have a foreseeable effect of causing death may also be culpable. This prohibition applies also to health care professionals, and it may be argued that it is particularly strong in their case, since vulnerable patients have been entrusted to their care. It is thus clear that carers must never intend the death of their patients.

The situation in palliative care is further complicated by the fact that there are times when death appears to be a benefit, both from the patient's and the carer's perspective. Yet the carer is not permitted to intend it. At the same time, patients and carers wish to permit the use of medication to alleviate distress, even when this may have a foreseen effect of shortening life. In order to permit this, the doctrine of double effect is used.

This complex and controversial doctrine draws a distinction between intended and foreseen consequences, as is normal practice in health care where the benefits of treatments are intended, whereas the burdens and risks are foreseen but not intended. Heavy sedation in palliative care is seen to have a 'double effect': one effect is that which is intended for the relief of suffering, and the other is one which is foreseen but not intended, and this is the potential to shorten life. Thus the doctrine permits the relief of suffering by the only means possible, despite the fact that it is known that life may be shortened as a consequence of that treatment.

The doctrine presupposes that it is always possible to have a clear and unambiguous identification of the relevant intention. We feel that as technology advances and doctors have ever-increasing ability to sustain life artificially, even in a limited form, it is becoming increasingly important for doctors to be both clear and honest about their intentions, even though this may at times be difficult. For example, some would argue that disconnecting a respirator in those hopelessly ill or stopping artificial feeding for those in the persistent vegetative state is an act of intentionally shortening life. We would prefer to regard such acts as the intentional withdrawal of artificial means of prolonging life so as to permit death from natural causes. We accept that this distinction is difficult, but its admitted difficulty casts doubt on the usefulness of the doctrine of double effect.

Further discussion regarding the distinction between what we intend and what we foresee is contained in the section on withdrawing and withholding life-prolonging treatment in Chapter 13.

The doctrine of double effect is used by those who wish to maintain an *absolute* prohibition against the intentional shortening of life. If one does not hold that there is such an absolute prohibition against shortening life, then the doctrine of double effect with its attendant complexities is simply not necessary in palliative care. Those who prefer this position would simply state that the benefits of relieving distress may sometimes outweigh the harms of short-ening life when the patient is terminally ill. The advantage of this view is that it avoids the complex arguments surrounding the validity of distinctions between intending and foreseeing effects of one's acts, and it also seems to accord with the moral intuitions of most people. Common sense has a part to play in health care ethics, and this is one example where it is very important. Ordinary reasoning and moral intuition lead to the conclusion that the effective relief of suffering in terminal illness may sometimes justify the use of measures which entail a risk of shortening life.

Whilst the doctrine of double effect is sometimes used in health care ethics, it is not recognized in law, because in law people are taken to 'intend' the foreseeable effects of their actions. However, there is a special rule for the use of drugs which may hasten death which achieves virtually the same effect when it applies. Such drugs may be used where the patient is already dying, the drugs used are 'proper medical practice', and the 'motive' is to relieve pain (R v Adams 1957).

5.3.2   Acts and omissions

It is sometimes suggested that one bears a greater degree of account-ability or responsibility for the consequences of one's actions than one's omissions. In palliative care this becomes translated into a moral distinction between withdrawing treatment (an act) and with-holding treatment (an omission).

Morality is much more complex than this. Whether a decision leads to an act or an omission is not necessarily a morally relevant factor in its justification. In palliative care we are accountable for the process and partially for the outcomes of our decisions whether those outcomes are the result of an act or an omission. For instance, it may be morally wrong not to use artificial hydration, just as it may be to use it, depending on the circumstances. Moral justification rests on whether the care given or not given is appropriate to the patient's wishes, physical condition, and related factors.

Carers sometimes feel that it is easier to withhold a treatment than to withdraw it once started, and this applies particularly when the treatment may sustain or prolong life. Carers feel less causally responsible and therefore less blameworthy for something they did not do as opposed to something they did do. This has led to a reluctance to start treatment because of the moral difficulty of stopping it if it is ineffective, or if it becomes excessively burdensome in comparison to its benefits as the disease progresses. Carers feel more accountable for events caused by withdrawing treatment than for events which ensue when that treatment is withheld. This is illogical, but understandable.

Nevertheless, the fact is that in palliative care we are morally and legally responsible for our omissions as we are for our actions. Many life-sustaining and life-prolonging procedures are available, just as many options for symptom control are available. We are responsible for our choice—that is for choosing some options and discarding others. If a moral distinction is made between withholding and withdrawing treatment, for instance artificial hydration, and it is deemed potentially more blameworthy to withdraw treatment than to withhold it, then two adverse consequences ensue.

First, doctors become unwilling to start treatment when it is appropriate, in order to avoid stopping it when it is no longer appropriate. This can result in undertreatment of patients. Secondly, doctors become unwilling to stop life-prolonging treatment when it is no longer appropriate, because this constitutes a withdrawal of treatment which is seen as potentially blameworthy, particularly as it may contribute to the patient's death. This can result in overtreatment.

It is therefore not logical or helpful to make a moral distinction between withholding and withdrawing treatment. Clinical situations in palliative care change, often rapidly and unpredictably. It is important that treatment options are reviewed frequently, and that treatment appropriate to the present circumstance is given.

5.3.3 Killing and letting die

Medical technology has made it possible to prolong life much beyond the point at which death would naturally occur. It can now be said that many people die at the time they do because technological interventions have been withheld and they have been allowed to die of their illnesses. This is termed 'letting die'. It is permitted and is regarded as morally justified. Indeed it is morally required when the burdens and risks of life-prolonging treatment outweigh the benefits of those treatments for a particular patient.

Many people want to die without much intervention when they know that they are terminally ill, and those who die at home do not have access to intravenous fluids, cardiopulmonary resuscitation, intravenous antibiotics, and other life-sustaining or life-prolonging manoeuvres. Thus letting die in some health care circumstances, and particularly in palliative care, has to be permitted.

On the other hand, society has an interest in prohibiting intentional killing (usually called murder) in all but exceptional circumstances such as war. It can be argued that because of the extent of patient vulnerability in the carer–patient relationship, there are overwhelming reasons for maintaining society's strong prohibition of killing in this relationship. In other words, killing may be something that doctors and professional carers, even more than others, should not do.

Unfortunately, the advent of technology has made the distinction between killing and letting die very blurred in many cases. It is difficult to maintain that the act of switching off a respirator is killing as opposed to letting die. It can and should be argued that the patient then dies as a result of overwhelming illness and not because the respirator was turned off. It is contrary to common sense to say that anyone who withholds or withdraws life-prolonging treatment from terminally ill patients is causally and morally responsible for their death, because without such treatment the patient would have been dead due to overwhelming illness. Similarly, the person who has to ration renal dialysis is not held morally responsible for the death of patients not treated.

The reality is that:

1. in an increasing number of cases the distinction between killing and letting die is difficult to draw, but

2. society needs to maintain its prohibition against killing in order to protect its members, whilst

3. letting die has to be permitted, for instance when the burdens and risks of life-prolonging or life-sustaining treatment outweigh its benefits.

In order to achieve 2 and 3 the vast majority of societies prohibit active euthanasia, and permit letting die where the burdens and risks of treatment outweigh its benefits or where the competent patient refuses treatment.

It is important to note that the distinction between killing and letting die cannot be simplified into a distinction between an act and an omission, and even if it could we have established that such a distinction alone could not provide the moral justification of a decision. There are some situations in which letting die cannot be justified, even in palliative care. This is reflected in law; failing to act where one is legally bound to act is culpable in law, and if the patient dies as a result of such a failure it would be homicide.

A more detailed discussion of this topic is included in Chapter 13, p. 270.

5.4   Formal guides to clinical decision making

Clinical decision making is a complex and difficult matter. In order to try to assist doctors to make 'better' decisions, a number of initiatives have been tried. These include formal guides to clinical decisions such as flow charts, clinical guidelines, and protocols, and more complex models such as clinical decision analysis which incorporates the patient's valuation of various outcomes in a branching sequence of events and choices to form a flow chart which resembles a tree.

The four-principle system of approaching health care ethics, as described in Chapter 1, was intended as a way of assisting professionals to see all morally relevant aspects of a clinical problem by assessing it with regard to the principles of respect for autonomy, beneficence, non-maleficence, and justice. Whilst conflicts between the principles prevent this model from providing solutions for the clinician, it is still a useful checklist in difficult situations where the principles act as signposts in the moral aspects of decision making. The system gives guidelines on the process of decision making, but does not dictate which decision is 'right' in the clinical situation.

A second source of intended assistance in decision making is the formal guides, such as flow charts and clinical guidelines (Hurwitz 1998). They have been introduced for two reasons; firstly in order to create the greatest likelihood of achieving what is considered by health care professionals to be the best outcome for patients, and secondly to provide the most cost-effective treatments for a population. It is vital to differentiate between these two goals. The second will be considered in the chapter on resource allocation. Moral problems concerning the use of such guides in decisions regarding the individual patient have already been mentioned (pp. 21, 111), and will be further considered here. It is assumed for the purposes of discussion that all treatments in the guides are available within the allocated budget, although we appreciate that this is often a gross oversimplification of the real-life situation.

Formal guides so far used in palliative care have been relatively simple flow charts or algorithms, which are intended to direct treatment along the lines of current opinion of 'best practice'. Possible events are drawn in a progressive manner, so that decisions are made in a step-like fashion following a pathway indicated by arrows. One management decision option only is suggested following each specified event. Since only one management manoeuvre is given for each event, choice is largely eliminated by this type of aid.

The act of following a flow chart leaves no room for consideration of the preferred treatment or outcome for a particular patient, because it is designed to impose what is thought to be best practice for the majority of patients. This could mean either the management which is thought to be most cost-effective or that which gives outcomes which 'the average' patient would value most. In either case there is no opportunity for the patient to exercise choice based on personal values and priorities, or for the doctor to act or give advice to further the total good of this particular patient. As previously stated, the slavish following of flow charts or other clinical guidelines fails to respect the autonomy of both physician and patient, and is contrary to the philosophy of palliative care. Such formal guides should be used only as aids to decision making, and the exclusive use of such rigid instructions in palliative care would be unethical. The guides are related to the *science* of medicine, which is concerned with generalities, rather than the *art* of palliative care, which is concerned with particularities and is based on practical wisdom or *phronesis*.

Clinical decision analysis is a more sophisticated tool which is being developed in the sphere of general medicine. It is designed to aid decisions concerning individual patients and so it incorporates quality of life evaluations of the various outcomes. These evaluations are reached by the particular patient. The probability of each outcome is incorporated into a mathematical assessment of the overall value of a treatment by multiplying the quality of life assessment by the probability for each outcome. The result is a complex and time-consuming diagrammatic representation of all treatments and their overall value or 'utility' to the patient. The treatment chosen is then that with the greatest numerical result on the utility assessment.

Practical problems abound with regard to the use of this model in palliative care, not the least of which is a high degree of uncertainty about the probabilities of various outcomes, the exhaustive nature of questioning for the patient, and the necessity for the patient to contemplate all possible outcomes, many of which could be very unpleasant.

The major moral problem is that the decision is ultimately taken entirely by the doctor alone, and this is compounded by the fact that this decision is based on a mathematical calculation of doubtful validity in palliative care where the probabilities of various outcomes are extremely uncertain. It is also impossible for the patient to elect to take a risk. Outcomes which cannot be measured and represented numerically do not feature in the decision-making 'tree', and so some important personal goals which should influence the decision are likely to be omitted from the calculations.

There is a more sinister moral consequence inherent in the exclusive and indiscriminate use of formal guides for decisions making. Where treatment is chosen on the basis of a flow chart or following clinical guidelines, the carers may be seen to have discharged their professional responsibility for that decision simply by following the guidelines. There is a danger in a litigation-conscious environment that professionals may be tempted to evade legal and moral accountability for individual decisions by claiming that their only responsibility is to follow the guidelines, no matter how inappropriate the resulting course may be for a particular patient. Indeed, it will require some courage to act contrary to guidelines, especially if it proves more costly, and doctors will have increasing difficulty in justifying decisions which accord with the patient's good but fall outside the guidelines. Moreover, if an adverse outcome ensues after a decision made according to the guidelines, the professionals may feel that they have no clinical responsibility for it.

Formal aids to decision making should be used only as aids in palliative care, and not as rigid rules. Our task as professionals is to offer and deliver treatment appropriate to our particular patient, and treatment suggested by following a formal aid may be inappropriate. In palliative care our professional responsibility is not discharged only by following guidelines because that responsibility relates to individual patient care.

5.5 Conclusions

1. The moral quality of a clinical decision is dependent on the process of that decision and not only on the outcome. We are accountable and responsible for the way in which our decisions are reached.

2. In palliative care outcomes are multifactorial and unpredictable. Therefore, we are usually only partially responsible in a causal sense for the outcome, and are blameworthy or praiseworthy in respect of the outcome only to the extent that our decision did of itself influence the outcome.

3. Since our understanding of the problem from a whole person perspective will always be limited, good communication and acceptance of the patient's views is essential in reaching the desired goal of a consensus decision.

4. Treatment cannot be imposed on the competent patient who refuses it. Professional carers cannot be forced to give treatment which they strongly feel is contrary to the patient's good, the latter being based on a benefits to burdens/risks calculus.

5. A decision in palliative care may result in an act or an omission; either may be blameworthy or praiseworthy. We are morally accountable for the outcomes of our omissions to the same extent that we are for the outcomes of our acts. There is no moral difference between withholding and withdrawing treatment.

6. Letting die is permitted in certain circumstances whereas killing is prohibited. The doctrine of double effect which relies on a moral distinction between intended and foreseen events allows the use of measures to relieve suffering even though they carry a significant risk of shortening life. The doctrine is not necessary for moral justification of symptom relief at the end of life.

7. Rigid adherence to clinical guidelines denies respect for patient and carer autonomy, and may prevent the pursuit of the patient's total good.

6

Giving information

Where is the Life we have lost in living?
Where is the wisdom we have lost in knowledge?
Where is the knowledge we have lost in information?
                    T. S. Eliot, *The Rock*, Pt 1 (1934)

God be in my mouth,
And in my speaking.
                    Sarum Missal (11th century)

How much of the truth should be told, and to whom? 'Patients should be told as much of the truth as they want to know.' This simple statement sums up current teaching in palliative care and health care generally in the United Kingdom, North America, and Western Europe. Yet it is not universal practice to follow this recommendation, since carers still often tell relatives the news about diagnosis and only then consider 'whether the patient should be told'. Furthermore, it is naive to assume that even if all professionals did follow this principle, all the moral dilemmas surrounding truth-telling in palliative care would be resolved. This simple principle, whilst justifiable and necessary in clinical practice, is not a sufficient answer to all our problems.

We have chosen to divide the difficulties of giving information into two sections, the first dealing with information about the diagnosis and prognosis of the illness, and the second with information about different treatments. In the next chapter we shall discuss the related issues of confidentiality.

It is important to be clear about the moral justifications for our initial principle. Recent documents about patients' rights proclaim that all patients have a 'right to know' about their illness and available treatments. What is the moral foundation of this 'right'?

First, and most important, is our fundamental belief in the value of truth. Human beings live in communities, and since our ability to sustain a community life depends on honest communication, a very high value is placed on truth and honesty in our dealings with each other. The high value which we place on truth in community, in conjunction with our concept of individuality and of ownership of our bodies, leads to the conclusion that we are entitled to the truth about our health which intimately relates to our welfare.

A second justification derives from the first and applies to the patient–carer relationship, which we have said is fundamentally dependent on trust. If either party fails to be honest, the aims of this relationship are unlikely to be achieved. If health care staff in general are not honest with patients, the fundamental relationship of trust in patient–carer relationships is undermined.

A third justification rests on the need for information in order to enable patients to make genuine choices about treatment. It is important to stress that this is not the primary moral reason for telling patients the truth. The truth is of value in itself, and not just as a means to the end of participation in decision making by patients.

It is also sometimes claimed that the aim of health care (and therefore of palliative care) is to increase patient autonomy, and if this view is accepted, then it follows that patients should be told everything that they can possibly comprehend in order to maximize their autonomy in making choices. This would entail giving all patients large amounts of information which they do not necessarily want. Since we do not consider that increasing autonomy is the aim of palliative care, we do not feel that trying to give all patients the 'whole truth' for this reason is justified.

6.1 The professional responsibility

If we uphold the principle that we ought to tell the truth in palliative care, we are still left with many questions. Are there some choices the professional must make and for which moral responsibility must be taken, such as how much of the truth to tell, or how to tell it? We can consider first the question of the need for professional choice and therefore moral responsibility in deciding how much of the truth to tell.

It could be argued that there are two positions which minimize moral choices by the professional. First, there is the position that patients must be told all the information they can comprehend, and secondly the position that the professional's task is limited to giving only that information which patients indicate that they want.

In answer to the first proposal that patients should be told as much of the 'whole truth' as they can comprehend, we have already said that there would be serious adverse consequences as a result of giving large amounts of bad news. Patients would be told all possible outcomes including ways of dying. Many of these possible outcomes would never actually happen to the particular patient who would have been unjustifiably traumatized by such information, much of which would turn out to be irrelevant. In any case, limitations of time and attention span render this proposal totally impractical.

The second proposal suggests that the professional answers the patients' questions truthfully but only, and always, literally. It is sometimes said that the patient should be in control of the flow of information, by being allowed not only to ask questions but also by being asked how much information they really want. This is done in order to enable patients to gain knowledge at a pace at which they can assimilate it, and in order to respect their wishes. It should not be done simply in an attempt to avoid taking moral responsibility for judging exactly what aspects of the truth should be told. Unfortunately, although initially attractive, this proposal is an oversimplification of the situation and some examples help to illustrate this.

In some circumstances where patients have indicated that further bad news is not wanted, doctors and nurses may feel that they should be told more about the illness for their 'medical good'. For instance, if a patient with carcinoma of the breast and also neck pain is found to have bone metastases in the cervical spine, with a risk of cord compression and quadriplegia, then a hard collar should be worn and the patient should try to avoid falls, etc. It may even be advisable for the patient to rest pending radiotherapy in order to minimize the risks of quadriplegia. In this situation the patient has to be given the 'bad news' of cervical metastases in order to adjust lifestyle patterns to minimize the risk of the very serious harm of quadriplegia. Thus circumstances may arise in which the professional becomes aware of major risks of serious adverse consequences which can be averted by informing the patient who can then cooperate to minimize those risks and consequences. The professional does have to make a moral choice in this situation, and in fact has no alternative but to make such a choice. The possible courses of action are to:

1. tell the patient only the information which is being requested, and hope adverse events will not ensue, or

2. inform the patient of the bad news, even though it is unwanted and unwelcome, so that the adverse event can be avoided, or

3. suggest that if further bad news is unwanted, the patient may wish to pass decisions to the professional who may then give advice about lifestyle, etc., but without unwanted explanation regarding the underlying disease progression.

It is obvious that if the adverse event does ensue, the patient will inevitably become aware of the gravity of the situation, and will probably also come to realize that professional knowledge which was withheld from them might have averted the event if it had been passed on. On balance, it seems most important to use professional knowledge to try to avoid serious harm to the patient. In other words, options 2 and 3 above seem preferable to option 1.

From this discussion it is apparent that the professional, in deciding how much of the truth to tell, has to make a moral choice which involves a harms/risks to benefits calculus relating to the impact of the information on the patient. Such a calculus is obviously difficult, and getting it right for a particular patient is very much part of the art of palliative care. It is clear that if the patients' total good is our aim, and if their medical good, which is a major component in their total good, can be served only by our passing on to them our professional knowledge, then we must take moral responsibility for sharing the necessary aspects of that knowledge with them. A decision not to give any information not requested by the patient purely to avoid such responsibility amounts to moral abandonment. Thus sometimes professionals in palliative care are morally obliged to give more information than the patient actually requests, based on a harms/benefits calculus which is undertaken on the basis of professional knowledge and experience.

Is it ever appropriate to give less information than the patient is asking for, following a harms/benefits calculus, or in other words to withhold knowledge which the patient is requesting? At first sight the answer to this question would seem to be 'no', because we have suggested that patients are entitled to the truth about their illness. In some clinical situations the morally appropriate course of action may seem less obvious.

For example, if we see a patient who is clearly cachectic, lethargic, and extremely ill, and who we consider probably has at most two to four weeks to live, and the patient asks if survival of three years is likely, we may rightly conclude that the patient is unaware of the seriousness of the situation, and we may further postulate that a degree of denial may be contributing to this lack of awareness. In view of the probability of some denial, we may try to reduce the amount of information given at this time by replying that survival of three years is *very unlikely*, rather than saying truthfully that we can say with reasonable certainty that it is *impossible*. In this case it may be morally defensible to give less than the bare truth to the patient, based on a harms/benefits calculus.

It must be said, however, that whenever less than the whole truth is given in reply to a direct question, the burden of justification for withholding information lies heavily with the professional. This accords with our view that professional carers do have to make choices about how much of the truth should be told at a particular time, and must take moral responsibility for that choice.

It is important to stress that it is extremely difficult to justify lying to patients. Therefore, a general rule prohibiting lying to patients is morally appropriate. By lying we mean telling the patient something we know to be false in order to deceive the patient. It is obviously very hazardous to lay down absolutely binding moral rules for behaviour. On the other hand, we have been unable to find a clinical example where lying to a patient can be morally justified, nor could a general rule of permitting lying to patients, even in their own interests, have beneficial consequences for society in general. In our dealings with patients we should not in general intend to deceive them, nor should we tell them information we know to be false in order to do so.

This is not to say that the 'whole truth' (as far as we can know it) has to be given at a particular time; we bear responsibility for our decision regarding how much of the truth should be given at a particular meeting with the patient, as illustrated in the preceding example relating to the likely length of future life.

6.2   Whom do we tell?

When a group of health care professionals are asked who should be given information about the illness, virtually all will reply that the patient should be offered information first, and yet in practice this still does not happen (Wilkes 1989). Why is this so, and is the practice of telling relatives the diagnosis before the patient ever morally justifiable?

It seems that many carers still feel that it is easier to tell the relatives first, presumably because they find telling the family and facing their distress easier than telling the patient and then facing his or her possibly greater distress. This is not a valid moral justification for the practice of telling relatives the diagnosis first, because the purpose of palliative care is not and never has been to minimize distress to the carer. The professional carer's feelings in this regard are not morally relevant. This may seem a hard thing to say, but it needs to be said if the patients' right to the truth is to be upheld. In Chapter 3, p. 68, we discuss whether professionals have an obligation to give relatives information about the patient's illness.

Sometimes carers consider that they need to ask the relatives' opinion of the patient's best interests before deciding what to tell the patient and we discuss this issue later. Alternatively, carers may consider that the relatives' wishes should rightly influence what the patient is told. In fact, if we consider that the competent patient is entitled to the truth, then the wishes of the relatives in the matter are hardly, if at all, morally relevant.

If, however, the patient is unconscious or confused and is therefore unable to assimilate information, then the next of kin should be informed of the seriousness of the situation provided that the patient has not previously requested that information be withheld from them. The relatives are informed in order to explain the patient's medical situation and to enable them to prepare themselves for the future. They may also be involved in the patient's care at home, and therefore need to understand the medical situation. When the patient cannot benefit from being told the truth, and indeed may be harmed because of being able to retain only frightening and disconnected partial truths, then the family who can benefit from the knowledge should be told. This is permissible because the patient in this situation is not competent to authorize professionals to explain the medical situation to the family, and it seems from clinical experience that few patients object to their loved ones being informed in these circumstances. Carers therefore assume that incompetent patients would consent to knowledge about their medical circumstances being shared with close relatives.

6.3 The influence of relatives

Most of the difficulties surrounding disclosure of the diagnosis and prognosis to competent patients arise as a result of suggestions from the friends and relatives that information should either be withheld from the patient, or more rarely should be given when the patient is reluctant to receive it. There is much confusion still about the moral and legal basis for influence by the relatives in this matter, and therefore great confusion arises when clashes occur between the patient's and the relatives' views on what information should be given to whom.

In fact it is the case that competent patients are entitled, both morally and legally, to information from the professionals about their illness, and that those professionals have a moral and legal responsibility to judge how much of the truth to tell and how to tell it at a particular time. It is clear that relatives do not have a legal right to determine what information the patient is given. Nevertheless, professionals often feel that relatives have a moral right to have their wishes respected in this regard, even if they conflict with those of the patient. Why should this be?

It must be admitted that the relatives can be intimidating to the professionals in comparison with a frail, exhausted, anxious, and vulnerable patient. It is obvious that intimidation by relatives is not a good moral reason for withholding information from the patient, or indeed for forcing unwanted information on the patient.

Sometimes when relatives have been told the diagnosis in advance of the patient, they voice the opinion that the patient should not be told the diagnosis and/or the prognosis. Various explanations may be suggested for this, but fundamentally the basis for this view is always either the interests of the relatives themselves, or their perception of the patient's best interests, or sometimes a combination of both. When this situation arises, it is helpful to enquire from the relatives why it is they feel that the patient should not be told; this not only helps to enlighten the carers about important family relationships, but also may give some indication of the relatives' view of the patient's personality and previous ways of coping with crises.

Examples of the relatives' interests reveal that they are not necessarily purely self-seeking. For instance, a loving spouse may not want the patient told the diagnosis because he or she thinks that the patient may then give up hope, and may then die sooner, leaving the spouse to grieve sooner. The basis of this self-interest is love, even though it may appear a little misguided to others. Sometimes relatives simply feel that they cannot face the patient's distress when the diagnosis is revealed, and they therefore would prefer the patient to remain in ignorance of it. More often the relatives explain that they feel that it is not in the patient's best interests to know the diagnosis, perhaps because of previous depression in response to life crises, or because they think that the patient will simply give up and therefore suffer an earlier death, perhaps having declined active treatment. However, withholding information usually entails disadvantages to the patient.

For example, a frail man with known bone metastases from a carcinoma of the breast was due to see his surgeon for a routine out-patient appointment. On the day when he was due to go, results of recent blood tests became available, and they indicated that it was likely he also had liver metastases and he was anaemic. In order to ensure that this information was passed on to the surgeon, the patient's daughter was informed of the results by phone. However, she asked the surgeon to withhold information about the likely liver metastases from the patient, and he agreed. The result of this was that the patient was denied the opportunity to discuss the likely progress of the illness with the surgeon. Instead, the patient gained the mistaken impression that a blood transfusion was likely to be of considerable benefit, and he then expected this to be arranged. It was necessary later to withhold transfusion when further investigation revealed hypercalcaemia, very extensive liver metastases, and a pleural effusion, which together made it very unlikely that he would gain symptomatic improvement from transfusion. The patient's daughter afterwards said that she had intended to tell the patient about his blood test results after the out-patient appointment with the surgeon, but this policy effectively denied the patient the oppor-tunity to talk about the true state of his illness with the surgeon. We do not think that professionals should agree to withhold information from patients at the request of their relatives and prior to seeing the patient. Moreover, it is clear that informing the relative of an important investigation result rather than telling the patient first is a breach of confidentiality and may lead to subsequent adverse con-sequences for the patient, and perhaps also the relative.

In other circumstances relatives may want the patient to be informed. For example, a young wife with two children whose self-employed husband is showing reluctance to be told that he has a terminal illness may want him to be informed against his wishes in order that he may make some provision for her and her children. This example of self-interest is not primarily selfish either. Does the young man in this case have a right to remain in ignorance of his illness? We are not thought to have a right to remain in ignorance of our bank overdraft or of a state of war relating to our nation, because we are members of a community to which we have responsibilities.

Rarely, relatives may suggest that a reluctant patient should be informed of the seriousness of the situation in order that treatment requiring consent can be discussed and commenced, or that an appropriate lifestyle can be adopted.

In all of these examples, there is a difference between the patients' and the relatives' perception of the amount of the truth which should be disclosed, and to whom. It should be noted that while it is common for relatives to suggest that information be withheld from the patient, it is rare for them to suggest it be withheld from themselves!

It is clear from our earlier discussions of the aims of palliative care that the good of the patient is paramount, and it is not morally justifiable to sacrifice it to the good of the relatives. This is true even if the good of the relatives may seem in some way greater. It is true because of the fundamental aim of palliative care. Therefore, the patient's good should be the first consideration of the professional in disclosing information, and the patient should not be exposed to possible harm for the sake of furthering the relatives' interests, however understandable and loving they may seem.

In the first example, the loving spouse usually finds emotional separation from the patient who does not know the diagnosis very painful, and gentle explanation about the merits of open communication between them, together with reassurance that knowing the diagnosis will not necessarily result in earlier death, is usually sufficient to make the spouse concur with honesty between the professional and the patient. Similarly, most relatives do understand that their own fear of facing the patient's distress when the diagnosis is revealed is not a moral reason for refusing the patient information.

It is clear in these simple but common examples that it is not morally justifiable to withhold information from the patient because of the relatives' interests.

On the other hand, the issue of giving information to a patient (who is reluctant to receive it) in the interests of relatives is more complex because it involves our ideas of the human being as a member of a community as well as an individual. This essential connection is made clear in the concept of autonomy; an autonomous person is one who is self-governing and has regard for the needs of others when determining his own actions.

The example of the young man who prefers to avoid knowledge of the terminal nature of the illness, where his wife feels that in the interests of the whole family he should be made aware of it, illustrates this problem. As an individual, we may say that the patient can make the choice not to be informed about his illness, but as a member of the intimate community of a family it would seem that he does not have a moral right to insulate himself against crises which involve that whole family, and that therefore he should be given some indication of the seriousness of the situation. The problem arises in the first place because his wife was told the diagnosis instead of the patient, but this is likely to happen when the patient initially declines information. Several courses of action are available to the professional as follows:

1. The patient is told that his condition is very serious, is potentially life-threatening, and that he should bear this in mind in running his business affairs. The doctor takes responsibility for making the decision to tell the patient this much on the basis of the patient's total good as a family member. The argument against this is that the doctor alone cannot know the patient's total good, which is dependent on the patient's perceptions of the situation.

2. His wife may be asked if she would like to tell him of his condition, perhaps when a doctor or nurse is present if she wishes it. Since his wife is already in possession of the information, and has intimate knowledge of her husband's feelings, it seems justifiable to ask her if she would like to be the one to tell him. This course must not be adopted simply to 'let the doctor off the hook'. It is justifiable only if the doctor feels that the patient should be given further indications of the seriousness of his condition, and if further contact with the doctor for more information is assured.

3. If the patient remains adamant that he wishes to know nothing about his condition because he does not want 'bad news' but wants to concentrate on positive belief that all will be well, then the doctor may decide not to give him further information at this point on the grounds that he is probably exercising a substantial degree of denial and the harms of interfering with this may outweigh any benefits to the patient, and indeed to the family.

In fact, most people with children have a strong sense of family commitment, and unless fixed in denial will want some information about the seriousness of their condition in order to cater for family needs.

For instance, it is often necessary to point out to patients that weakness has decreased their mobility to such an extent that two people are needed to lift them, and that one elderly spouse, however determined and loving, is simply unable to do this alone. Occasionally, it may also be necessary to explain to the patient some fears which the spouse may have but may feel unable to discuss with the patient, usually because of associated guilt and shame. Fears of the sight of blood, of a dead body, or of seeing someone vomit or choke are all well known, and even though they may seem irrational, they are very real. Indeed, their irrationality makes them difficult to abolish by explanation or reassurance. Since patients are members of the family community, they cannot and should not be shielded from the reality of the family situation, for to do so would be to regard them as less than autonomous and to accord them less than the respect which is their due. It is not appropriate to treat patients as though they are young children simply because they are terminally ill.

A more extreme example of patients' responsibilities to relatives and the community arises from the potential for harm caused by spread of the HIV virus. Patients who are known to be HIV positive are not considered to have a moral right to remain in ignorance of their HIV status, because of the very serious damage which can be inflicted on others if they behave as if HIV negative when they are in fact infected with the virus. This example illustrates clearly that there is no absolute right to remain in ignorance of serious illness regardless of the consequences to others.

Relatives caring for a patient in their house may go so far as to refuse carers access to the patient unless an undertaking not to disclose the diagnosis is made; they may do this for their own interests or because of their perception of the patient's interests. The carers then have a choice of whether to collude with the relatives in withholding information, in order to gain access to the patient to relieve symptoms, or they may refuse to be coerced in this way by the relatives and leave the house, in which case the patient does not receive the much-needed help.

In this situation it is usually worth calling the relatives' bluff by adopting the latter attitude and offering to leave; most families will then acquiesce to help from the professionals, especially if assurance is given that the patient will be told only the amount of detail about the illness which is requested or which is required in order to alleviate symptoms. It may of course also be morally justifiable under such coercion from the relatives to agree not to disclose the diagnosis in order to alleviate symptoms, if one judges from the available evidence that the patient's greatest need is relief from physical distress. This moral dilemma is rare, but unfortunately it still occurs.

It is important to appreciate that the relatives have no moral or legal right to refuse to allow the patient to be given information in accordance with the professional's judgement, but they do have the legal right to refuse the carer access to the house. As a last resort, a legal procedure to remove the patient to a 'place of safety' can be instigated.

In the vast majority of cases, with explanation and persuasion relatives permit access and care in accordance with the patient's wishes, but it is important that professionals are always aware of the moral and legal perspectives in this difficult situation. Whilst one must always listen to the relatives' reasons for not wanting the diagnosis disclosed to the patient, the health professional's responsibility is still to serve the patient's good as previously described.

In summary, the relatives' interests do not constitute a morally justifiable reason for withholding information from the patient, if the professional judges that the patient should be informed. In contrast, it is sometimes morally justifiable to give patients information which they have been reluctant to receive in order to serve the relatives' interests and those of the patient as part of the family. Whilst patients have a right to the truth, they do not have an absolute right to be shielded from the reality of a situation which affects not only themselves but also their close family who are often participating actively in care. This was illustrated in the example of the self-employed young man with a wife and children. The fact of being terminally ill does not mean that a competent adult escapes the degree of moral responsibility for the welfare of others, especially close family, that we all bear.

6.4 How the truth is told

Professional carers are obviously morally responsible for the way in which they communicate the truth to the patient and family. Much has been written about the practical skills involved, and we have stressed the importance of appropriate attitudes in palliative care.

The practical skills include an ability to give information so that the patient can assimilate it, understand it, believe it, and interpret it in the context of their own lives. Unfortunately, despite our best efforts, and especially when anxious and frightened, patients may find it difficult or impossible to assimilate, understand, and interpret information and may also be unable to believe it. Professionals have a moral responsibility to take advantage of the increasing knowledge about effective communication strategies, and to use those skills together with their natural abilities to do their best for each patient. The importance of giving time for discussions to be repeated, or of using tape-recordings of discussions, is now recognized. Nevertheless, the nature of human beings is such that perfect communication of complex and often frightening information to patients is not likely to be possible. We are therefore striving for an adequate level of understanding on behalf of the patient, regarding the diagnosis and prognosis and also treatment options with their associated benefits, risks, and harms.

It has to be said that in palliative care it occasionally happens that patients are simply unable to believe very bad news, and react by effectively denying it, sometimes with disastrous results. Despite our best efforts, it seems impossible to prevent this. Patients may also hold false beliefs about their illness or treatments, despite persuasion using reasoned argument by the carers.

For example, a young woman with a carcinoma of the breast which appeared clinically to be confined within the breast refused surgery because she believed that surgical intervention would so upset the natural balance of her body's defences that she would die of the tumour anyway. Despite radiotherapy and hormone treatment the tumour grew and many times caused life-threatening bleeding. After a complete collapse following one such bleed she asked for surgery. When asked why she had changed her mind and if she was now sure she wanted to proceed with a major cosmetic but non-curative operation, she said that she had never previously believed the tumour would kill her, but having been near to death she now did believe it and wanted surgery to avoid fatal haemorrhage. She died of metastases after an extensive operation, having forgone an earlier and possibly curative operation because of what most people would regard as a false belief, which she held despite reasoned argument. In this case the information was assimilated, understood, and interpreted, but was not believed.

It seems that even appropriate attitudes, natural ability, and all the communication skills we can learn cannot prevent such occurrences. We are morally required to try to persuade patients by reasoned argument to pursue a course of action which we believe to be very beneficial, but ultimately we may not be able to alter a patient's fixed beliefs or inability to believe. If the carers have done all they can to enable the patient to assimilate, understand, and interpret information, have tried to persuade patients to undergo treatment which they believe to be beneficial, and they have done so with compassion and respect, then they cannot be held blameworthy on account of the consequences.

6.5 Standards of disclosure

In addition to information about the diagnosis, patients require details of available treatments to combat the illness itself, or to relieve symptoms or alleviate psychological distress. The issue of disclosure, especially when related to informed consent, has many legal implications and has been much discussed in the courts. We are concerned primarily with the morality of disclosure, but some of the possible standards for disclosure are interesting and discussion surrounding them has contributed to public debate on this matter.

The first standard for doctors is that of 'professional practice', that is the traditional practices of a group of physicians. This is the only legal standard in the United Kingdom. This standard acknowledges the professional task in selecting how much of the truth should be told, but it fails to take into account the special needs of a particular patient (which the physician may not know) or the fact that the standards of professional disclosure may not be morally adequate. The second is the 'reasonable person' standard which is the amount of information a hypothetical reasonable person would require. This comprises the facts that most people consider relevant and essential when making a similar treatment decision. The problem is that there is no general common knowledge of this list of facts for every condition and circumstance, so it is a difficult standard to apply, and it does not take account of a particular patient's needs. The third is the subjective standard which is the information that this particular patient requests. This acknowledges the particular patient's needs, but not the carer's responsibility to pass on information which is believed necessary to ensure that the patient is adequately informed to make a decision.

Thus none of the above standards alone is sufficient as a moral guide to disclosure of information related to treatments. A simpler but more satisfactory guide can be deduced from our previous discussions about the mutual aims of carer and patient in palliative care and their roles and partnership in the decision-making process. Information which should be disclosed is:

1. that which patients usually consider relevant and essential in deciding whether treatment should be refused or accepted—in other words that which seems important to most people in the carer's experience or knowledge;

2. that which the professional believes to be relevant and essential or important. This may include the sorts of benefits, risks, and harms which may not generally be known to the public, or which the patient may not consider important until their relevance is pointed out by the carer, or information which the carer feels is especially relevant to this particular patient;

3. that which this patient requests and which has not been disclosed in 1 or 2;

4. the recommendation of the professional regarding treatment for this particular patient in this particular circumstance. We have maintained that the professional does have a duty to give advice based on knowledge and experience of the present and previous patients.

An example helps to illustrate the above points. A young nurse with metastatic breast cancer had been found to have cerebral metastases identified on brain scan, and the issue of whether cerebral irradiation was in her interests was being discussed. Following points 1 and 2 above she was informed that such irradiation might decrease her symptoms and prevent physical disability and loss of cognitive function, but that such treatment was not curative of the illness and did entail side-effects such as drowsiness, poor concentration, hair loss, and so on. Since this patient was a nurse, it was pointed out that radiotherapy treatment might decrease the requirement for steroids in control of symptoms. As an example of point 3 the patient then asked if she had single or multiple metastases on the scan, and if they were large or small, and her questions were answered. Following point 4, the consultant clinical oncologist advised this young woman not to undergo cerebral irradiation on the grounds that the harms and risks in her case outweighed the likely benefits, since her metastases were large and multiple and she had also indicated that the process of undergoing radiotherapy treatment would constitute a major burden to her.

Whilst the above list of information which should be given is useful and is an improvement on any one of the legal standards, some moral difficulties remain.

6.6   Moral difficulties in giving information

The first and perhaps the most obvious is the *uncertain* nature of information in palliative care. In other aspects of health care the percentage chance of many benefits, risks, and harms is generally known. For instance, the incidence of complications following surgical procedures is known, as is the percentage of patients showing some sort of response to chemotherapy in various cancers, or the average length of life with various degenerative neurological conditions. Research in the field of palliative care is fraught with practical and moral difficulties and as a result percentage responses to various treatments may not be known with anything like the same precision as in other areas of health care. Consequently, there is less 'hard' factual information about the generalities of disease behaviour and response to treatment in palliative care, despite the fact that many professionals are striving to increase our scientific knowledge.

In addition, whilst we may have some idea of what may happen to the average patient, we cannot extrapolate from this to produce a prediction of how this particular disease will respond in this particular patient. This serves to compound our initial fairly high degree of uncertainty.

Thus both patient and professional carer are faced with the problem of making decisions about treatment on the basis of what is known, when what is and can be known is very limited. The only morally justifiable course is to be honest with the patient about the degree of uncertainty regarding outcomes of treatment.

It is therefore necessary to explain to patients that certain treatments are more or less likely to cause a disease response or relieve symptoms, and similarly that particular side-effects are usual, likely, or uncommon, and that some risks are either frequent or rare. Patients should also be told what is likely to happen without treatment. It is then necessary for the professional to indicate his or her own recommendation in the particular circumstances. For instance, we know that opiates are very likely to relieve many pains, but that they are also extremely likely to cause constipation, often cause nausea which may be transient, and sometimes cause sedation which is usually also transient. At the same time we may advise the patient to try opiates because they are by far the most effective analgesics in the particular situation, and because side-effects can be controlled by other means.

An important moral consequence of this degree of uncertainty is that the professional should be willing to take a risk with treatment if the patient so wishes it. As described in the previous chapter, treatments with a small chance of a major benefit, and those with a small chance of a minor benefit but without overwhelming adverse effects, should be offered, even when the carer if in the patient's circumstances would not personally choose to accept the risks and harms entailed. The uncertainty of outcome means that patients must be permitted to take risks. On the other hand, if the professional knows that there is only a minor chance of a small benefit, for example a less than 20 per cent chance of a three months prolongation of life, with severe associated harms and risks for this particular patient, it seems to us reasonable for the professional to refuse to give the treatment to this patient.

A second moral difficulty concerns how the risks and harms of treatment should be *expressed*. The impact of a description of a certain benefit, risk, or harm on the patient depends in part on how that benefit, risk, or harm is expressed. For example, a palliative chemotherapy treatment may have a 40 per cent chance of causing some disease regression, with a 70 per cent chance of distressing side-effects and a 10 per cent chance of life-threatening infection as a result of marrow suppression. If the patient is simply told that it carries a 'good' or 'reasonable' chance of response, at the cost of some side-effects and with a low chance of infection, the patient is very likely to accept the treatment, particularly if their illness is terminal and they know that there is no other way of slowing the progress of the disease. If, on the other hand, they are told that this treatment has a 60 per cent (or greater than even) chance of doing no good at all, whilst still carrying a 70 per cent chance of causing distressing side-effects and a 10 per cent chance of a life-threatening infection, they will be much less likely to accept it. Risks may be perceived differently according to whether they are expressed in terms of disease or symptom response or non-response, or in terms of survival as opposed to death.

On balance, it may be best to try to describe the risks in both ways in order to try to eliminate this sort of selection bias. Many doctors know that they can influence the patient's decision by quoting risks and harms and benefits in different ways. What is important is that we try to give information so that the patient who wishes to take part in the decision is adequately informed to do so. Ideally, the greatest possible understanding should be attained, but this should not be achieved at the expense of harm to the patient. Information overload may actually decrease the patient's ability to make decisions, and the judgement of how much detail and how many statistics a particular patient is able to assimilate, understand, and use in the decision is a complex matter and is very much part of the art of palliative care. It is also a value judgement and so is part of the moral responsibility of the professional in palliative care.

A third moral difficulty relates to the degree *of participation* that patients wish in decision making; for each degree of involvement, there is an adequate level of information. In other words, the more fully patients wish to be involved, the more information is required to ensure that they are *adequately informed* to take joint responsibility for the decisions reached. Moral problems occur if there is disparity between the amount of information patients want and the degree of control they wish to exert over treatments given. Whilst all patients have a right to decline treatment for whatever reason, and even if they have declined information, they do not have a right to insist on a treatment, particularly if they have declined the relevant information.

Clinical examples help to clarify this difficulty. Sometimes a patient declines information relating to the seriousness of the medical situation, for instance irreversible intestinal obstruction due to malignancy, and so is in effect inadequately informed to make treatment decisions, and yet wants to participate in decisions by requesting that intravenous hydration and feeding are commenced and continued. This situation is uncommon but may occasionally arise in relation to life-prolonging or life-sustaining treatments where the patient is unable and/or unwilling to face the fact that life is ending. The solutions to this difficult and sensitive situation will be discussed in more detail in Chapter 7.

Patients are free to choose and must be permitted to choose the amount of participation that they want in treatment decisions. Some wish to be fully involved, and therefore require as much information as possible, others simply prefer to pass decision-making responsibility to the professionals, having given some indication of their own goals and values. The latter group frequently decline detailed information which should not then be forced upon them. What is important is that the patient is adequately informed for the degree of participation that they have chosen. The corollary of this is that patients cannot expect to assume joint responsibility for treatment decisions if they at the same time decline to be adequately informed.

The professional task entails ensuring that the information offered is adequate for the degree of participation that the patient has chosen. It is not morally justifiable for professionals to insist that patients participate fully in decisions; such a position would require that information be forced on patients in order to render them adequately informed to take joint responsibility for decisions. As we have said earlier, the aim of palliative care is not to try to increase patient autonomy in decision making.

What information could be construed as essential in order for patients to be adequately informed to participate *fully* in treatment decisions? Patients need to know:

1. the basic medical situation, which includes what is likely to happen with no active treatment;

2. the treatments which may be helpful in their case, including what is likely to happen if they undergo treatment. This includes the nature and likelihood of the benefits, risks, and harms entailed in the treatments offered;

3. the professionals' recommendation in their particular circumstances.

It is obvious that this amounts to a considerable amount of information. Many patients may either not want to try or not be able to assimilate, understand, and interpret it in order to participate fully in decision making. In this case they will not be adequately informed to participate fully, and whilst the professional will obviously take their views, based on their degree of understanding, into account, ultimately the professional must take most of the responsibility for the treatment decision. In other words, patients cannot insist on certain treatments if they have declined essential information or if they are unable to be adequately informed about their situation and/or those treatments. Thus the patient with irreversible malignant intestinal obstruction who declines to discuss the medical situation is not in a position to take responsibility for a decision to initiate or continue intravenous hydration and/or feeding. See Chapter 7 for a discussion on the morally acceptable solutions to this clinical problem.

We have said that the professional's recommendations with respect to treatment should be part of the information given, and that rational persuasion may sometimes be necessary to encourage a patient to accept a treatment. Neither of these equates with coercion or manipulation, which are not morally justifiable.

Coercion occurs where the carer intentionally uses a threat of harm in order to force a patient to adopt a certain course of action. For instance, a doctor may say that unless a patient in the palliative care situation agrees to undergo a certain drug treatment for symptom control, that patient will be denied access to the palliative care service in the future. Unfortunately, some patients have been told in the past that unless they accept a certain treatment, for instance radiotherapy for established malignant paraplegia, which carries only a small prospect of returning function to the lower limbs, they will be denied the nursing care which they need. Such a threat is obviously not morally defensible. It can be argued that in extreme life-threatening situations where a curative treatment is available and the patient declines it, coercion may be justified in order to cause the patient to consent to the treatment. By definition, this situation does not arise in palliative care.

More commonly, patients may be manipulated into making a certain decision. For instance, information which would be considered essential for an adequately informed decision may be omitted (such as the risks and harms of drugs, chemotherapy, or radiotherapy), or the likelihood of success of a treatment may be exaggerated, or in very serious cases a lie may be told to the patient. These strategies involve intentional deception of the patient and are not morally defensible.

The very many moral difficulties of giving information in the palliative care setting have been described. They illustrate that such disclosure necessarily involves very difficult moral choices which entail complex benefits versus risks and harms analyses and a very great degree of uncertainty. The combination of these factors means that carers should guard against taking too rigid a moral line when judging the degree of disclosure which colleagues consider to be appropriate. Others, including patients and their relatives who do not have our professional knowledge and experience, may not share our opinions or may need time to form their own opinion which they may change as the course of the illness and response to treatments becomes clearer. The moral and practical complexities surrounding the disclosure of information mean that a great deal of practical wisdom, or *phronesis*, is required to achieve the aims of palliative care in relation to this issue.

6.7　Conclusions

1. Patients should be told at least as much of the truth about their illness as they wish to know.

2. Patients do not have an absolute right to remain in ignorance of aspects of their illness which have a major impact on their family, professional carers, or the community.

3. The professional task sometimes entails giving information on the basis of a harms/benefits analysis to patients who may not be requesting it.

4. Carers are morally responsible for giving information sensitively and should take advantage of whatever has been learned about effective communication.

5. Patients choose the extent to which they wish to be involved in decision making; for each level of involvement there is an appropriate and necessary understanding of the facts related to the illness and treatments which is required in order to be adequately informed.

7

Confidentiality

*I would tell them of my own intention to keep counsel ...
and I will venture to recommend them, as an old-Parliamen-
tarian, to do the same.*
W. E. Gladstone, *Hansard*, 7 June 1896

7.1 The moral basis for rules of confidentiality in palliative care

It is generally accepted that there is a moral right to control access to
one's own body, and also to information about oneself. This is called
a right to privacy. What is the moral basis for this right?

Firstly, privacy is essential for the development of fundamentally
important human relationships such as friendship and love. Secondly,
privacy may be considered to be derived from respect for autonomy,
which requires that others do not act against one's choices regarding
access to one's body or to personal information. Neither of these
provides sufficient justification for the privacy which we feel that
non-autonomous patients should still be accorded. For instance, we
do not consider it right for unconscious or confused patients to
be left physically exposed, nor for the bodies of deceased patients
to left visible to all, nor for information about non-autonomous
or deceased patients to be generally divulged. Therefore, a right to
privacy must also be related in some fundamental way to human
dignity. It seems that we are so made that we consider that all human
beings, whether autonomous or not, are worthy of some fundamental degree of privacy. (We acknowledge that some members of
the press and media may not hold this view, but they are exceptional
in their attitudes to information transfer.)

Secondly, patients grant access to their bodies and personal information to professional carers on the implicit understanding that
such access and information is to be used for the patient's benefit.
Respect for autonomy demands that information be used in accordance with the patients' wishes. Fidelity to the promise implicit in
the patient–carer relationship demands that the carer adheres to the

publicly accepted codes of practice within that relationship. Thus the attitude of respect for autonomy and the moral principle of fidelity to promises both demand that patients should retain some measure of control over the information which carers hold about them.

Thirdly, rules of confidentiality may also be justified by their consequences. We have said that trust is essential in the patient–carer relationship. That trust would certainly be very much diminished if the carer considered that there was no obligation to respect the patient's wishes with regard to disclosure of personal information. Patients would very soon become reluctant to confide in professionals if they thought that the personal information disclosed would be divulged to others without their authorization. Thus there are good grounds for establishing fairly strict rules to prevent carers divulging such information without the patients' implicit or explicit consent to do so.

Such rules, called rules of confidentiality, have been present in medical ethics from the time of Hippocrates, and are well established in our current codes of practice for health care professionals. They state that carers may not divulge information that they learn about a patient in the course of their professional relationship unless that patient implicitly or explicitly consents to such a disclosure. These rules are not absolutely binding, and some important circumstances where they may justifiably be broken will be discussed later.

Confidentiality is said to be infringed if a patient discloses information in confidence to a carer, and that carer then divulges it to another person without the patient's permission. The information may be divulged intentionally or as a result of failure to protect the information adequately.

It is necessary to consider in more detail what constitutes information disclosed in confidence, with whom is it implicitly agreed that it may be shared, and what moral justifications there are for infringing confidentiality.

7.2 What constitutes confidential information?

Information may be regarded as more or less personal or private in its nature, according to its type and degree of detail:

1. Identification: name, address, date of birth, sex, occupation, marital status, etc. are all routinely collected by all health care

organizations and are accessible to a wide range of administrative, clinical, and often ancillary staff such as those providing 'hotel services' in hospitals.

2. Medical information: diagnosis or diagnostic-related group, extent of the disease and disability, results of investigations, treatment details, and past medical history including alcohol or drug abuse. This is generally known to medical, nursing, and paramedical staff, and also to administrative staff who process information.

3. Social information: family and social relationships, housing, finances, and occupational history. This is accessible to the same group of staff as medical information.

4. Psychological information: emotional state such as anxiety or depression, acceptance or denial of diagnostic information, marital, sexual, or family relationship problems, spiritual problems, etc. This is accessible to medical, nursing, and paramedical staff, and to the extent which it is recorded in the notes or discussed verbally it is also accessible to administrative staff who process information.

It is obvious that information of a confidential nature which is disclosed to only one or two members of the caring team is nevertheless accessible and may in fact be divulged to very many other people in the course of palliative care. It is also increasingly recorded on computerized information systems to which very many people not connected with the patient's care potentially have access. This leads us to our second question.

7.3   Sharing confidential information

Patients are aware that palliative care will be carried out by a *team* of staff, including administrative, clerical, and ancillary staff as well as nurses, doctors, and paramedical staff. With whom do they expect and implicitly agree that information may be shared? Can we presume that they agree to this information being shared among all those who have access to it?

Whilst patients probably agree that information in levels 1, 2, and 3 above needs to be shared by medical, nursing, and paramedical staff such as social workers, physiotherapists, and dieticians, and whilst they may accept that administrative staff such as secretaries and ward clerks also have access to this information, they may be less happy about general dissemination of psychological information within the team. Ideally, patients should be asked if they are happy about information being given to those who need to know it in order to offer the best care. In fact we tend to assume in palliative care that patients have agreed to the sharing of all levels of information within the team. This assumption is based in part on a second assumption common to patients and carers: that all members of the team are bound not to divulge the information outside the context of necessary communication within their professional role.

If we suggest that patients have not implicitly agreed to the sharing of psychological information with all members of the team, then who should be made aware of it? Obviously, staff whose role in the patient's care necessitates or would be facilitated by certain knowledge should be given that knowledge. This is called divulging information on a 'need to know' basis and is generally considered to be morally justifiable. Such staff may be described as those who 'must know' and those who 'should know'. A list will obviously include doctors, nurses, and paramedical staff involved in the patients' care, but others such as complementary therapists, clergy, and volunteers may also need to be told relevant information in order to do their job effectively. For instance, an aromatherapist may need to know if a patient is anxious or unable to relax, a clergyman will need to be aware of spiritual anxieties, feelings of guilt, and relationship problems, and volunteers administering drinks or sitting with confused patients may need some medical information such as the existence of diabetes, or factors which tend to induce anxiety or relaxation.

It must be acknowledged that the team approach to palliative care, in which regular team meetings are held where all the patients' problems are discussed, tends to result in all members of the team knowing all that is known to other members about the patient. The end result of this practice is that all information is effectively shared. It is not reasonable to assume that patients agree to this.

It is therefore morally preferable to share very sensitive information, such as patients' sexual difficulties, previous drug or alcohol abuse, or HIV status, only with those members of the team who must know and who should know it. If information may be regarded as sensitive, team members should ask the patient's permission before sharing it with colleagues, and even then should divulge it only with those who need to know it. Obviously, patients' wishes in this regard should be respected, unless there are overwhelming reasons (as discussed later) for not doing so.

Sometimes nursing, medical, and paramedical staff need to discuss particular patients with *colleagues outside the team*, in order to gain advice or an informal second opinion. This can often be done without mentioning details which could identify the patient. If a more detailed and formal opinion is needed, the colleague will need all the relevant information as a basis for giving advice, and in this case the patient will be asked about such a second opinion and so has an opportunity to consent to or refuse the sharing of information.

It is obviously not morally defensible to divulge confidential information to colleagues frivolously, for instance at parties, when no possible benefit to the patient can result and when the patient has not consented either explicitly or implicitly to information being passed outside the team.

Health care workers in palliative care are frequently accompanied by other *trainees* at various stages of their studies. Where those trainees are not part of the caring team, patients should be asked if they consent to the trainee having access to confidential information. Patients' wishes should then be respected. Trainees should be reminded of rules of confidentiality.

Clinical staff in palliative care sometimes discuss patients about whom they are particularly concerned or distressed with their *spouses* or *partners*. This practice is probably not harmful provided that no information which could identify the patient is divulged. Many staff gain support from their spouses and partners, and it would be very difficult to justify and uphold a rule that they must never discuss clinical problems at home. What is important is that information which could identify the patient is not divulged.

Many patients seem to agree implicitly with the sharing of many aspects of information, particularly those relating to medical matters, with their close *relatives* and *spouses*. Nevertheless, it is not safe to assume that the patient does agree to disclosure. If relatives are told the diagnosis before a competent patient is informed, a breach of confidentiality of a serious nature has occurred. Even though many patients fortunately do not resent this because they wish their relatives to be informed, the professional carers are not morally entitled to disclose this information to the relatives without the patient's permission. For example, it is common for the spouse or grown-up children of the patient to ask for information about the prognosis of the illness, particularly in terms of time, that the patient has not asked for and does not know. Health care professionals often breach confidentiality by providing such information to relatives; indeed, such breaches of confidentiality are so common that many health care professionals are either unaware of them or have come to consider that the relatives are entitled in some way to this information. The situation is further complicated by the fact that the patient can hardly give consent to the sharing of this information because the patient is unaware of the information itself. A breach of confidentiality by giving information to relatives without the patient's consent requires justification. There are some circumstances where infringement of confidentiality by divulging some information to relatives is morally justified, and these are discussed later.

7.4   Disclosure of information to third parties

Whilst *relatives* are not entitled to information unless the patient gives consent, in practice the vast majority of patients wish their spouses or partners, and often their parents or children, to be informed of the medical facts of their illness, and they usually give consent very readily for this information to be shared.

Psychological information is, however, another matter. Patients often wish to talk confidentially to carers about deeply personal matters such as close relationships, spiritual problems, or unresolved issues in their past life, as well as their present feelings associated with the illness. Such information should not be passed on to relatives unless the patient indicates that this is permitted. For instance, it is obviously inappropriate to pass on accounts of marital difficulties, or anxieties about the spouse's ability to cope, to the patient's spouse unless permission to do so has been given. Frequently such information is of such a sensitive nature that it is inappropriate to divulge it to any other carers unless the patient requests this. Alternatively it may simply be irrelevant to the task of palliative care, and therefore there may be no need to pass it on to any other team members.

Close friends of the patient may ask for medical details, but disclosure about this or social or psychological aspects of the patient's condition constitutes an infringement of confidentiality which requires justification. Such justification is usually possible only if the friend is closely involved in the patient's care.

The social services or other community *service agencies* may request information. It is reasonable to pass on those facts which such agencies need to know, since they are part of the caring team. One exception is financial information. Government bodies cannot expect professionals to pass on financial information; such information must be given directly by the patient to those authorized to collect it. For instance, entitlement to services free of charge is often based on a 'means test' which entails disclosure of the patient's financial circumstances. The patient should pass on this information directly to those whose responsibility it is to deliver and charge for such services.

Lawyers acting on behalf of the patient may sometimes need to ask doctors about the patient's testamentary capacity. The patient's permission should be sought. Difficult moral dilemmas arise where patients have become disorientated, forgetful, or confused and the doctor feels that their mental state is sufficiently clouded to cast doubt upon their testamentary capacity in respect of writing a will. In this situation it can be argued that the doctor is morally (and perhaps legally) obliged to inform the lawyer that the patient is not competent to make a will. Of course it can also be argued that if confused to such an extent, the patient is not competent to give or withhold consent for information relating to testamentary capacity to be divulged.

Occasionally in palliative care the *press* may come to hear of some incident in the life of a patient which they feel should be reported in the public interest, or which they feel would generate sufficient public interest to sell newspapers. The palliative care team have no moral right to divulge information about a patient to the press. Indeed, since whatever is divulged to the press is likely to be widely disseminated, if not also seriously distorted, it can be argued that those involved in palliative care should *never* divulge information to them, unless the patient has specifically requested that this be done and has issued precise instructions as to what should be said. Unfortunately, the press may attempt to coerce palliative care staff to disclose information by measures such as threatening to try to extort the story from the patient's relatives or other sources, or by maintaining that at least the story will be factually correct if the doctor gives the information as opposed to the reporters obtaining it piecemeal from other sources. Such attempts at coercion are morally indefensible and must be resisted. It is also obviously morally wrong to accept a bribe in return for selling confidential information to the press.

Very rarely the *police* may ask for information relating to a patient or to the patient's family. Such information should not be divulged unless the patient gives permission. Occasionally, if the safety of the patient or other members of society is at stake, breaches of confidentiality are justifiable and may in fact be morally obligatory. This is much more common in the field of forensic psychiatry than in palliative care, but some patients may become violent if confused or paranoid, and if third parties are thought to be at risk, the police should be given the minimum information necessary to prevent harm to those other parties. This is a justifiable infringement of confidentiality.

Health care staff outside the patient's caring team have access to much information via computer networks, especially in hospitals. This is a serious moral problem which is becoming all-pervasive as ever-increasing amounts of information are retained in this way for managerial purposes as well as to facilitate patient care. Those not directly concerned with the patient's clinical care, including managers, are not entitled to information which is identified with a particular patient. It is tempting for staff working in hospitals who know a patient socially to log on to the computer system to retrieve information. This is morally indefensible, even if it is motivated by concern for the patient. Those responsible for keeping computerized records are responsible for the security of the information. Unfortunately, breaches of security as just described are extremely difficult to discover or prevent. Therefore, there is a very strong moral case for limiting the amount of information held on computer, and for limiting access to whatever information is held. The Data Protection Act seeks to ensure that the confidentiality of records is safeguarded by law. The managerial advantages of holding clinical information about a patient on a computer do not justify greatly increased risks of breaches of confidentiality. Instead, the information that may be centrally held and whose security cannot be safeguarded should be limited by the requirement to respect patients' privacy in terms of their medical records. In other words, it should be the interests of patients and not primarily those of managers which dictate how patient-specific information is kept.

7.5   Confidentiality and the non-autonomous patient

Rules of confidentiality in palliative care are grounded partly on their necessity for the success of the patient–carer relationship, and partly on the privacy which is an essential component of human dignity. Thus these rules can be justified without recourse to the essential attitude of respect for autonomy in palliative care. Rules of confidentiality apply to non-autonomous patients and even to deceased patients just as they do to autonomous patients.

In palliative care there are many clinical situations where patients are no longer autonomous, such as when consciousness is diminished before death, or when brain tumours, dementia, or biochemical disturbances cause confusion. In these common circumstances patients are no longer able to give consent for confidential information to be divulged. In practice, information is given to relatives or close friends. What information is it morally permissible to disclose?

The team may be guided by the patient's previously expressed wishes in this respect. If these are not known, then it seems reasonable to explain the medical situation to relatives and close friends. If this is not done, serious harm in the form of distress due to ignorance about the causes of the patient's deterioration is likely to occur. Moreover, some medical information will have to be disclosed if relatives or friends who are caring for the patient are to do so effectively.

Psychological information may be disclosed only in order to prevent moderate or serious harm to relatives and close friends. For example, when a hypoxic patient who had always been unrealistic about her prognosis became confused, she developed paranoid ideas related to her closest friend whom she accused of stealing from her and of refusing to assist with care so that the patient could be discharged. Serious distress was caused to the friend, and explanation about the patient's medical condition, and her difficulty in accepting the diagnosis and the reality of her situation, was required in order to relieve that distress. Only the minimum amount of information necessary to alleviate the friend's distress was disclosed. On another occasion a patient who was somewhat confused became very agitated when members of staff looked at him through a window in the door of his room. The staff later learned that he had been a prisoner during World War II and his agitation was probably related to recollections of a prison cell experience. It was vital that the staff caring for him passed on this information to other carers, both lay and professional, so that his distress could be avoided. He was not able to consent to the transfer of this information about his psychological state.

These two examples are very different. The first describes a case where the interests of the friend point to disclosure. The second is a case where disclosure is in the interests of the patient. In law, disclosure of information regarding non-autonomous patients to friends, carers, or relatives is justified only if in the patient's interests, not if in the interests of those friends, carers, or relatives. However, it seems reasonable to argue that in some circumstances, for instance when the dying patient is comatose, it is morally justifiable to divulge some information to enable those close to the patient to prepare themselve for the patient's death.

It is important to stress that the duty of confidentiality is not dependent on patient autonomy, and so rules of confidentiality still apply where the patient is non-autonomous. Moral judgement is required on behalf of professionals to decide when confidentiality should be breached in the interests of the patient, relatives, or occasionally staff.

7.6   Justifications for infringements of confidentiality

The duty of confidentiality for health care professionals is not absolute, just as the right to privacy is not absolute. There are some exceptional circumstances where breaches of confidentiality are considered to be morally justifiable, and may indeed be morally obligatory. All of the justifications are based on the necessity to avoid possible and probable harm to the patient or others. The minimum information necessary to prevent this harm should be disclosed, and then only after proper consideration of the circumstances. Some examples of justified infringements of confidentiality are helpful.

7.6.1   *Prevention of harm to non-autonomous patients*

Where relatives or friends are caring for a non-autonomous patient they may need to know aspects of medical and psychological information in order to care effectively for the patient. For instance, it is obvious that they must be told about certain movements which could cause pain or even pathological fracture, they will need explanation of behaviour related to severe depression or of confusion related to biochemical disorders such as hypercalcaemia or inappropriate ADH secretion, and they may need explanation of paranoia which can result from a combination of fear, anxiety, and confusion. The non-autonomous patient cannot consent to this transfer of information, and so it is the moral responsibility of the carer to judge what should be disclosed on the 'need to know' basis.

Occasionally a confused and very ill patient may be cared for by a relative or friend who is either malicious or is incompetent to do so by reason of alcoholism, drug addiction, or mental illness. In order to prevent harm to the patient, confidential information may need to be passed on by professional carers to the police or social services in order that the patient can be removed to a place of safety.

7.6.2 *Prevention of harm to autonomous patients*

Competent patients may be asked if they consent to information being passed on to others. They should be told the precise nature of information which may be communicated to others. For instance, some patients decide that they do not want to know various details about their illness, and they can be asked if they want certain relatives or friends to be informed instead. If they consent, then by definition there is no breach of confidentiality in passing the specified information to those persons whom they have nominated.

Rarely it may be justifiable to pass on information about autonomous patients without their consent in order to prevent harm to those patients. One such example arises when a doctor completes a Social Services form to entitle the patient to a grant called the Attendance Allowance under the 'special rules' which pertain if the patient is believed to have less than six months to live. Patients who have chosen not to be informed of their prognosis may have their section of this form filled in on their behalf by a member of the professional team or by a relative. Their general practitioner, hospital consultant, or palliative care specialist fills in an additional form. These forms contain confidential information about the patient's diagnosis, previous, current, and proposed future treatment, and general condition, and this information is passed on to those administering the grant. Usually it is possible to ask the patient if one may communicate such medical details to the administrators, but very occasionally discussion of the conditions under which 'special rules' apply would inevitably lead to the patient being given information which had been explicitly refused. In this circumstance it is considered morally justifiable to pass on the information without the patient's consent in order to avoid traumatizing the patient with unwanted information.

Where patients are in residential care, either in a retirement or nursing home, they may sometimes refuse consent for their carers to be informed about their medical condition. If they cannot be persuaded to allow carers to be given information which the latter need to know, then exceptionally a breach of confidentiality may be justified in order to prevent harm to the patient. For example, if the patient is diabetic and at risk of hypoglycaemia the carers should know. Similarly, if the patient is in warden-supervised accommodation, the wardens may need to know about diabetes, epilepsy, severe forgetfulness, or confusion. If such information is disclosed, the minimum required for the patient's safety should be divulged.

7.6.3 *Prevention of harm to others*

Rarely in palliative care a professional may come to know that a patient has violent tendencies, perhaps related to paranoia, and if carers believe that there is a significant and unavoidable risk of serious harm to a third party then they have an obligation to try to persuade the patient to inform the third party. If the patient refuses to do this then the professional has a duty to breach confidentiality in order to prevent harm to the third party. It is then necessary to inform the person at risk and/or the police.

More commonly, moral difficulties can surround the issue of fitness to drive. Doctors who considers patients unsafe to drive and therefore a risk to others as well as to themselves have a duty to tell such patients that they must not drive. Medical reasons in palliative care might be sedation induced by medication, or hemianopia (serious visual disturbance) or epilepsy due to cerebral tumour. If such patients continue to drive, as occasionally they do, the doctor may feel justified or perhaps morally obliged to breach confidentiality and tell the vehicle licensing authorities who may then instigate further procedures to assess fitness to drive and may remove such patients' driving licences as a result. Such a breach of confidentiality is justified in order to prevent likely and serious harm to others as well as to the patient.

Where there is a probable harm to society, the law may require that information be disclosed and this is generally considered an adequate moral justification. For instance, notifiable diseases are reported in the interests of public health, and very rarely a judge may request disclosure of confidential information in the interests of preventing or solving serious crime. However, in law obligations to breach confidentiality are exceptional—there is no general duty to do so.

The complex issue of transfer of information regarding patients' HIV status has received much attention, and because of this we shall not rehearse the arguments in great detail. Suffice it to say that an HIV positive patient who transmits the virus to others poses a very serious threat of harm to those others. Most infected patients can be persuaded to inform their sexual partners of their HIV status and prevent such infection. Some patients refuse to do this. When a general practitioner has as his patients both the infected person and the spouse of that infected person, then that doctor may consider it justifiable to inform the spouse of the highly probable nature of the risk, and of the seriousness of the illness. We would consider that such a breach of confidentiality is justifiable. Others consider that the suggested adverse consequences of breaches of confidentiality related to HIV status, such as reluctance of potentially infected patients to attend STD clinics, outweigh the adverse consequences of failing to inform the partners of infected patients. It is not possible to prove that this is so.

In principle, when one considers that an individual is also a member of the community, it seems justifiable to breach confidentiality where there is a significant risk of serious harm to others. If the precise circumstances where this is morally and legally permitted were generally understood, then the trusting nature of the patient–carer relationship could be preserved, whilst at the same time preventing serious avoidable harms to other members of the community.

7.6.4   Disclosure in the interests of present and future patients (research)

This is discussed in the chapter on the ethics of research in palliative care.

7.7 Conclusions

1. Everything that health care staff learn in the context of their professional relationship with the patient should be regarded as confidential.

2. Rules of confidentiality apply to non-autonomous and deceased patients as well as to autonomous patients.

3. Confidential information should be used only for the purpose for which it was given, and should not be passed on to others without the patient's consent unless necessary to avoid likely and moderate or serious harm to the patient or third parties.

8

Clinical treatment decisions

You do me wrong to take me out of the grave
Shakespeare, *King Lear*, Act 4, Scene 7 (*c.*1606)

'It's not very pleasant, though,' you may say, 'to have death right before one's eyes.' To this I would say, firstly, that death ought to be right there before the eyes of a young man just as much as an old one—the order in which we each receive our summons is not determined by our precedence in the register—and, secondly, that no one is so very old that it would be quite unnatural for him to hope for one more day ...

Seneca, *Letter XII* (*c.*AD 65)
(Translated from the Latin by Robin Campbell)

Patients and carers should have a shared awareness of the particular treatment considered. Whilst palliative treatments are given primarily either to prolong life or to relieve suffering or disability, the effects of many treatments are in fact mixed. For example, treatments given to prolong life, such as antibiotics for infections in AIDS, may also relieve symptoms by resolving the infection. Treatments given to relieve distress, such as analgesics, may prolong life by encouraging mobility and improved nutrition. In other cases, for example radiotherapy for superior vena cava obstruction, the aims of prolonging life and alleviating symptoms may be equally important.

8.1 Distinctions between medical treatment and care

It is common practice to divide health care activities into two groups, those providing what is considered to be *medical treatments* and those providing what is thought to represent *care*. A distinction is drawn between the two. It is then commonly assumed and stated that whilst medical treatments are always optional, care is always obligatory. The initial distinction and the assumption which follows have been used to provide moral justification for withholding or withdrawing life-prolonging activities classified as medical treatment, such as nasogastric feeding. It has been suggested that artificial feeding is not obligatory and so may be omitted or stopped *because* it is a medical treatment and not part of nursing care. We prefer to suggest that artificial feeding and other life-prolonging measures are not obligatory in palliative care, but not by reason of whether they may be considered medical treatment or nursing care. We do not consider that it is philosophically sound, practically helpful, or necessary to divide palliative care activities into these two groups and then make the assumption that medical treatment is optional and nursing care obligatory. Our reasons are as follows:

1.   It has proved extremely difficult to decide whether some activities such as artificial feeding via nasogastric tubes and gastrostomies constitute medical treatment or nursing care. Since the distinction is so difficult to draw, it seems unhelpful and perhaps impossible to use it as the basis for deciding whether an activity is obligatory or optional in a particular circumstance.

2.   Such a division encourages doctors and nurses to see themselves in two separate camps, because there is a general understanding that doctors are responsible for medical treatment, whereas nurses are responsible for care. This division of roles does not encourage professional partnership and teamwork. This is particularly so because the assumption that medical treatment is always optional but nursing is obligatory implies that doctors' activities may result in good or harm to the patient, whereas nurses' activities are necessarily good. Nurses come out white, whereas doctors may be white, black, or grey!

3.   It follows from the assumption that medical treatment is always optional while nursing care is obligatory that doctors' treatments may on balance be helpful or harmful but nursing care is always helpful and never harmful. Such a conclusion is obviously false, since there are many nursing care options available and each may be appropriate or inappropriate in a particular circumstance. Whilst it is acknowledged that the provision of care and indeed treatment *in general* is always obligatory, there is no *specific* care or treatment option which is always obligatory. It depends on the clinical circumstances.

For instance, the nursing care option of aggressive management of pressure sores involving debridement and desloughing is not obligatory when the patient is comatose and imminently dying. Indeed, it is probably obligatory not to provide such care in this situation, but instead to pursue the less aggressive options of a sophisticated pressure-relieving mattress and dressings involving minimal disturbance. Similarly, artificial feeding is not considered appropriate in this situation, and any consideration of whether it may best be described as a medical treatment or nursing care is simply irrelevant.

4. Whilst it is obviously morally obligatory to provide appropriate care in general for patients, it is also obviously morally obligatory to provide appropriate treatment. It is not acceptable to provide no treatment where some would be beneficial, any more than it is acceptable to provide no care where some would be beneficial. Confusion has probably arisen from the several meanings of the word 'care', which are dependent on the context in which it is used. It is obviously always necessary to be 'caring' in the sense of being concerned for the patient's welfare. It does not follow that all forms of care are appropriate or morally required.

In conclusion, even if it is possible to classify each activity as either care or medical treatment, the very fact of its falling into one category or the other is not relevant in deciding whether it is morally right or wrong in a particular case. We consider that it is preferable to take the view that *all* palliative care activities may be either appropriate or inappropriate.

8.2 Benefits to burdens/risks calculus

In Chapter 4 on clinical decision making we stressed that the *selection* of treatments which are offered to the autonomous patient, or considered by others on behalf of the non-autonomous patient, is dependent on the balance of their benefits against their harms and risks. This initial selection of treatment options is the moral responsibility of the professional team. Despite the difficulties of assessing the relative magnitude of benefits, burdens, and risks, and the uncertainty regarding the probability of each occurring in the particular clinical situation, this calculus is fundamental to the process of decision making.

When autonomous patients choose to be involved in choices regarding treatment, then the moral responsibility for the final treatment decision is shared; carers offer selected options which accord with the patient's medical good, and the patient makes a choice from these with the benefit of the team's advice. Some patients choose to pass decisions regarding treatment to professional carers, and those patients are responsible only for their refusal of or consent to the treatment advised by the team. In the case of non-autonomous patients, the responsibility for decision making lies with the professional team. The latter reach a conclusion on the basis of the patient's medical good and what they know from relatives of the patient's goals and values.

We have consistently maintained that trust and truthfulness underpin the carer–patient relationship, and honesty is morally required in describing the benefits, burdens, and risks of treatment options presented to patients. Benefits include psychological as well as physical gains, and may relate to prolongation of life or alleviation of distress. Burdens include the physical and psychological discomfort or inconvenience associated with the treatment, such as in-patient or out-patient hospital visits, taking tablets, having injections or infusions, and so on, as well as the known likely side-effects of drugs, for example nausea, constipation, and sedation. Risks are those serious harms which may occur as a result of the treatment, such as gastrointestinal haemorrhage from NSAIDs, or risk of shortening life if heavy sedation is used, or risk of prolonging life where this is considered undesirable (for instance by prolonging dying). Assessment of risk depends on both the likelihood and seriousness of the harm leading to a combined concept of overall risk. Only the patient can assess the overall significance of this risk according to his or her own perspective.

Uncertainty makes it difficult for us to be precise in our estimations of the likelihood of the benefits, burdens, and risks of a treatment for the particular patient, and it is appropriate for us to be honest about this uncertainty. Indeed, it is wrong for us to imply that we have more certain knowledge than we in fact possess. The personal significance of those benefits, burdens, and risks is assessed by the patient.

Obviously it is not practical to describe all the burdens and risks entailed in each treatment option; one solution is to try to give that information which a 'reasonable person' would consider material to the decision, plus any additional information which is thought to be particularly relevant to the patient, and to answer any further questions honestly. Patients rarely wish to be fully informed in so far as this is possible. Patients and carers together achieve a degree of understanding which they agree constitutes adequate information for the amount of participation in decision making that the patient requires.

For example, most patients do not want a detailed discussion of all the possible benefits, burdens, and risks of taking NSAIDs for bone pain; however, risks of gastrointestinal disturbance and haemorrhage are potentially serious and relatively common so that they become significant factors in decisions regarding use of these drugs. Therefore, patients who wish to be involved in making decisions are warned about them. In contrast, other side-effects of NSAIDs are either less common or less serious and so are not usually described in detail. Professionals cannot possibly pass on to patients all the possible burdens and risks of treatments. They therefore bear responsibility for making difficult decisions regarding the amount of information which each patient requires according to their chosen degree of participation in decision making.

8.3   Obligations and options in treatment decisions

The benefits to burdens/risks calculus provides the professional with guidance as to what treatments ought to be offered to the autonomous patient or considered for the non-autonomous patient. The 'ought' refers to the moral obligation to offer or provide a particular treatment in the clinical circumstances. Sometimes the balance may indicate to carers that they 'ought not' to offer or provide certain treatments.

Professionals have a moral obligation to provide treatments which carry a favourable balance of benefits to burdens or risks. If the balance is very favourable, for instance most uses of analgesics or simple life-sustaining medications such as insulin, then it would be considered obligatory to offer those treatments to the autonomous patient with appropriate advice, and it would also usually be considered obligatory to give such treatments to the non-autonomous patient. In many circumstances the balance of benefits to burdens or risks is not overwhelming in either direction, and in such cases the treatments are regarded as optional. The caring team together with the patient (or with the benefit of information about the patient's likely wishes obtained from the relatives) make a decision on the merits of the particular case. Finally, treatments which have only a minimal chance of benefit but which in the particular case entail overwhelming burdens or risks should not be provided. It could be said that such treatments are wrong and ought not to be provided, or that there is an obligation not to provide them.

For example, in most circumstances treatment measures such as analgesics, laxatives, and anti-emetics to relieve distressing symptoms, or rehabilitation to increase mobility, insulin for diabetes, diuretics for heart failure, and encouragement to eat and drink with the provision of food supplements are considered obligatory, and so they are provided unless the competent patient refuses them or they are clinically inappropriate, for instance if the patient is imminently dying. Other procedures such as stents for renal failure, antibiotics for pneumonia, and intravenous hydration are considered optional, so that carers will discuss whether they are or are not appropriate in each case. In contrast, cardiopulmonary resuscitation (CPR) and ventilation are not given to patients who are considered to be in the terminal phase of an incurable illness, and most palliative care specialists would consider it obligatory not to instigate CPR in such circumstances.

These examples illustrate that in each set of circumstances encountered in clinical practice we divide treatments into three categories, those which *ought* to be provided, those which are *optional*, and those which *ought not* to be provided. It is important to note that it is the balance of benefits to harms in the *particular clinical circumstances* which determines which category a treatment falls into—the treatments themselves are not intrinsically wrong or right.

The terms 'ordinary means' and 'extraordinary means' have in the past been used to classify treatments into two groups; extraordinary means were those that might be considered excessively invasive or burdensome, costly in terms of human or financial resources, or complex and perhaps 'unnatural'. In contrast, ordinary means were those considered to entail reasonable burdens or risks, costs, and complexity, or perhaps to be 'natural'. The terms 'extraordinary' and 'ordinary' did not mean 'unusual' and 'usual' respectively. The classification was used to determine which treatments could justifiably be withheld or withdrawn. We consider that the terms themselves are too vague and their use is too confusing for them to be helpful now in the discussion about life-prolonging and life-sustaining treatment.

Whilst autonomous patients can choose the extent to which they wish to participate in treatment decisions, those who are non-autonomous cannot participate in such decisions. Moreover, relatives cannot bear the legal or moral responsibility for treatment given, and therefore cannot in law consent to or refuse treatment on behalf of the patient. Therefore, professional carers have to bear the moral responsibility for making decisions on the patient's behalf. This responsibility cannot be passed to the relatives or to the state, however desirable these possibilities may seem. If an advance directive exists, then certain treatments may be refused or requested in certain circumstances, but it should be noted that the legal effects of refusals and requests are quite different. In addition, relatives may be able to enlighten carers about the patient's own values and may be able to give an opinion as to what the patient may have wanted in the circumstances. Knowledge of the patient's likely wishes assists carers to choose from the treatment options those which accord with the patient's own values and priorities.

8.4   Life-prolonging treatments

The moral problems which arise in palliative care regarding treatments intended primarily to prolong or sustain life relate to the balance of the benefit to the patient of the life prolonged compared with the burdens and risks of treatment. Whilst great value is placed on life by our society, and the lives of patients are entrusted to health care staff, those staff do not have a duty to try to preserve life at all costs.

'Quality is more important than quantity'—this statement has almost become a cliché in palliative care. Sometimes the quality of patients' lives artificially prolonged in the context of terminal illness is very poor, so that patients and carers may not consider extension of that life to be a benefit, or may consider that its benefit is outweighed by the burdens of treatment. Following the benefits to burdens/risks calculus in each case, staff consider that there are some life-prolonging measures which ought to be provided, some which are optional, and some which ought not to be provided. The moral 'ought' depends on the particular circumstances, and is derived from the benefits to burdens calculus.

Treatments which we consider ought not to be given in the circumstances are usually not offered to the autonomous patient (and are not discussed with the relatives of the non-autonomous patient). This is because it seems unhelpful to mention a treatment one is not prepared to provide. Those treatments considered optional or those which it is thought ought to be provided are discussed with the autonomous patient, and a consensus decision is reached in accordance with the patient's own values. If the patient is non-autonomous, optional treatments are given if it is thought that they accord with the patient's own values and priorities, and those which it is thought ought to be provided are given to the patient unless the latter has declined them via an advance directive.

This raises two important questions:

1. In what circumstances is it morally justifiable for professionals not to offer life-prolonging or life-sustaining treatments to autonomous patients?

2. What morally justifiable criteria should be used to decide which life-prolonging or life-sustaining treatments should be given to non-autonomous patients?

8.4.1 *In what circumstances is it morally justifiable for professionals not to offer life-prolonging and life-sustaining treatments to autonomous patients?*

This important issue is likely to become increasingly contentious with the rise in emphasis on the role of patient autonomy in health care choices. It was discussed in general terms in Chapter 4 on clinical decision making. There we took the view that so long as professionals are held accountable for giving treatments, they must have some choice whether or not to offer and administer those treatments. In other words, if the carers' autonomy is to be respected, they must be able to veto certain treatments which they feel do not accord with the patient's good. We feel that this course of action is preferable to the alternative option of offering all possible treatments and then indicating those we would not be prepared to give because of an adverse balance of benefit to harm in the particular patient's case.

Some examples may help to clarify the situations in which available treatments are not offered. The possible moral justifications for this practice are discussed.

Treatments considered futile

The most obvious example of a treatment not offered because professionals feel it is futile in the palliative care setting is cardiopulmonary resuscitation (CPR). This example is also relatively uncontroversial. We do not offer patients in the terminal phase of illness CPR, because it is extremely unlikely to be successful. It is exceedingly unlikely to achieve the desired physiological aim of restoring life because of irreversible organ failure. Moreover, patients could in some ways be harmed by it since attempted resuscitation is definitely understood by most to represent anything but a peaceful and dignified end!

It has sometimes been argued that treatments which the professionals consider futile should occasionally be given for two possible reasons: firstly to 'give patients hope' or secondly because the patients want to try them, perhaps because they feel they want to pursue every possible way of prolonging life. Patients may want to do this because life is very precious to them, but others are simply terrified of dying and will opt for any treatment which may put it off.

In the first case we consider that the practice is not defensible because the hope is false hope, and the practice entails colluding with the patient in this false hope by giving the treatment. Such collusion is basically dishonest, and so runs contrary to the essential requirements for truthfulness and trust in the patient–carer relationship.

In the second case we do not consider that the carer should provide the treatment because of the professional nature of the carer's relationship to the patient as described in Chapter 2. The carer has a professional responsibility to provide those treatments which accord with the patient's good by achieving medical benefit, and not to provide those which do not. It may be argued that giving the treatment benefits the patient simply by satisfying a desire to try it, but the professional task is not simply to do what the patient wants regardless of medical benefit. Since virtually all treatments entail some burdens and risks, overall harm is bound to result if there is no counterbalancing benefit. The professional does have a responsibility not to cause overall harm to the patient. If the patient is afraid of death, then those fears should be addressed and any reassurance possible should be given; providing a futile treatment will not benefit the patient in this situation. On the contrary, it may harm the patient physically and it may deter them from accepting what help can be given in dealing with fears surrounding death.

Therefore, we consider that on balance it seems morally justifiable not to offer treatments which the carers believe are physiologically futile.

Treatments whose burdens and risks greatly outweigh benefits

A more contentious question is whether carers should offer treatments which have a reasonable chance of achieving their intended physiological benefit, but where the value of that physiological benefit is considered to be greatly outweighed by the risks and burdens of the treatment.

An example in the palliative care setting concerns the ventilation of patients with respiratory failure due to motor neurone disease. In the United Kingdom this treatment is generally not offered or undertaken, whereas in North America it frequently is. What is important for our discussion is that in the United Kingdom the treatment is not offered.

The major reason for this, apart from resource constraints, is that the burdens of ventilation itself, which entails endotracheal tubes, periodic suction, and long periods in hospital, and the risks of infection and accidents (especially in the home setting) are considered to outweigh the benefit of the treatment in sustaining life in this situation.

The problem with the professionals making this decision is that it could be said that the only person who can assess and balance the various benefits, burdens, and risks is the patient. On the other hand, if the professionals are unwilling to give the treatment because, on the basis of their knowledge and experience of this particular patient as well as others, they consider that the burdens and risks of the treatment are overwhelmingly greater than the benefits, then it seems reasonable to suggest that they are justified in not offering the treatment. Once again there seems little point in raising the patient's hopes by mentioning a treatment, only to dash them again by explaining that the burdens and risks are so overwhelming that the carer is not willing to provide the treatment.

In this situation, not offering a life-prolonging treatment seems justifiable if and only if the professionals consider that following a benefits to burdens/risks calculus they would be unwilling to give the treatment. If they would be willing to give it to a competent patient who understood the benefits, risks, and burdens, then it should be discussed with such a patient.

Treatments which are not considered to further the patient's medical good

There can be several ways of dying of an incurable illness. Treatments which prevent death from one illness-related cause may succeed in prolonging life so that much more unpleasant and possibly terminal events ensue. Palliative care practice in some circumstances is about trying to manoeuvre the illness along the least unpleasant course and about enabling the patient to die of their illness in the least unpleasant way. How much choice should we give patients in determining as far as possible the course of their illness and the events from which they may finally die?

This issue is highly contentious. The simple answer seems to be that we should offer all patients the chance to determine the course of their illness and which terminal events they would prefer to cause their death. What would this mean in practice? Examples help to illustrate such problems in the palliative care setting, and consideration of them enables us to arrive at some solutions.

Tumours of the head and neck can prove fatal by causing asphyxiation, total dysphagia, catastrophic haemorrhage from the carotid artery, or pneumonia. Mercifully, many patients just seem to fade away and it is very difficult to identify a specific physiological cause of death. If a patient develops dysphagia, and tube-feeding by gastrostomy is undertaken, then that patient is likely to live long enough to develop either tracheal obstruction or haemorrhage. Similarly, if tracheostomy is undertaken, or resuscitation after severe haemorrhage is performed, then the patient is likely to live to develop dysphagia or to suffer recurrent haemorrhages, one of which is likely to prove fatal.

A similar situation occurs in locally advanced carcinoma of the cervix. This tumour commonly causes death by renal failure consequent upon bilateral obstruction of the ureters by tumour. Death can be prevented, at least for a while, by the insertion of small tubes called stents into the ureters to keep them open. The procedure is not excessively risky or unpleasant, and is usually physiologically successful in that renal failure is averted. The problem is that the patient is then likely to live long enough to develop a vesico-vaginal fistula (between the bladder and vagina), so that urine leaks from the vagina constantly, or a recto-vaginal fistula (between the rectum and vagina) so that faeces leaks through the vagina. Both of these fistulae are extremely unpleasant; the distress of a recto-vaginal fistula can be alleviated by an operation providing a defunctioning colostomy, but there is no really effective solution to the problems of a vesico-vaginal fistula.

If any of these life-prolonging treatments is offered it seems that the patient requires information about all these consequences, which mainly comprise ways of dying, in order to be adequately informed to participate in the decision. In other words, if a competent patient is to be offered a life-prolonging procedure, the medium- and long-term consequences of undergoing as well as of not undergoing the treatment should be explained. This will necessarily entail a rather gruesome discussion about ways of dying.

Many patients may well not want or welcome such a discussion, and in their case it is probably preferable and morally justifiable for the carers not to offer the treatment if in their professional opinion it will not further the patient's medical good because worse ways of dying are likely to ensue. In not offering the treatment the carers effectively make the decision on the patient's behalf. This seems unavoidable if the patient does not wish to be adequately informed to make the decision, because to be adequately informed entails a discussion about ways of dying. Such a patient is not competent, and does not wish to be rendered competent, to make the decision. In this situation it seems necessary and morally justifiable for the team not to offer life-prolonging treatment which they consider will make the course of the disease more traumatic, especially when the patient has a terminal illness and death is not too far distant, as is often the case in palliative care. Sometimes it seems possible to gain some indication of the patient's wishes with regard to life-prolonging treatments without a full discussion; the risk of this is that the patient is not fully informed and therefore cannot formulate ideas of his or her own best interests, so that an invalid conclusion may be reached by all.

Where patients have indicated that they want full participation in making decisions, life-prolonging measures which are not physiologically futile and whose intrinsic burdens and risks are not overwhelmingly greater than their benefits should be offered and discussed fully.

Treatments which are not considered to further the patient's total good

Lastly, and even more difficult, is the question of whether carers should offer treatments which have a reasonable chance of achieving their physiological aim, without causing burdens or risks excessive in relation to their benefits, and where more unpleasant terminal events are not likely to ensue, but the carers believe that for other reasons the quality of the life prolonged will be unacceptably poor. The quality of life may be poor for medical, social, or psychological reasons.

Medical reasons are factors related to illness which cause a poor quality of life. Such factors would include pain or other symptoms which are difficult to control without unacceptable side-effects, distressing immobility such as paralysis due to motor neurone disease or cord compression, or those causing distress in other ways such as inability to speak (dysphasia), offensive dressings, discharges, or fistulae. In these situations it may at first seem morally justifiable not to offer life-prolonging treatment.

For example, it may seem justifiable not to offer to treat pneumonia with antibiotics and physiotherapy if the patient is totally paralysed, dysphasic, and uncomfortable, or suffers the indignity of an major offensive dressing or discharge. It may seem reasonable not to offer ureteric stents to the woman with a vesico-vaginal fistula and nerve compression pain due to carcinoma of the cervix, and not to offer gastrostomy feeding to the patient who has disfigurement and bleeding from a tumour of the head and neck.

The problem with not offering life-prolonging treatment in such situations is that the only person who can really assess the quality and/or value of the life prolonged is the patient. In the above examples the patients are already experiencing the factors which could severely compromise their quality of life, and so they are in fact in a position to judge the value of continued life to them. Therefore, if patients are competent to decide whether in their present circumstances they would value continued life, then life-prolonging treatments should be offered even if it seems to the carers that their quality of life is poor. This is because assessment of quality of life is this situation is valid only if done by the person living it. Moreover, some people would still want life, and consider it valuable, even if its quality was poor.

For example, a mother with young children will often accept life which she and others would consider to be of poor quality, because she knows that it is of great value to her family and therefore to her. Young women in this situation as a result of advanced malignant disease tend to be tenacious of life and want it prolonged in order to give them more time with their families. Similarly, young mothers with AIDS may want to pursue active treatment to sustain life even when its quality appears poor to others.

It is important not to assume that we can assess another's quality of life, or the value of that life to them.

The same can be said where the patient has existing social or psychological problems which appear to cause them severe and continuing distress. Such patients should be offered life-prolonging treatments if they are competent to make a decision about whether the quality and value of their life is such that they want to pursue treatments to sustain or prolong it. A more detailed exploration of the concepts of quality of life and value of life is provided in Chapter 14.

Treatments not available due to resource constraints

Resources for health care are limited. Whilst most people consider it most unsatisfactory that considerations of resource allocation should influence decisions at the bedside about life-prolonging and life-sustaining treatment, it is true that some of these treatments, whilst technically possible, are not available because of lack of resources. Moreover, the carers are aware of resource constraints and may well feel that those technological resources which are available but very limited, for instance mechanical ventilation on intensive care units, or renal dialysis, or liver transplants, should be given to those patients who are likely to benefit most from them. This would definitely not include those already terminally ill. This does seem morally justifiable, even though it may be undesirable. This controversial issue is further discussed in Chapter 12 on resource allocation.

Summary

In summary we might say that it is morally justifiable not to offer life-prolonging and life-sustaining treatments to autonomous patients in the following circumstances: when they are physiologically futile, where their burdens and risks greatly outweigh their benefits, where they may prolong life so that much more unpleasant events which the patient declines to contemplate or discuss are very likely to ensue, and when the combination of resource constraints and justice require that the treatment be given to patients likely to derive more benefit from it. Not only should such treatments not be offered, but there is also a moral obligation not to provide them.

In contrast, we should offer all those life-prolonging and life-sustaining treatments which we described as obligatory or optional. Optional treatments are those which carry a good or reasonable hope of achieving their physiological aim without entailing excessive burdens and/or risks and which accord with the patient's medical good. Even if such treatments carry a low chance of achieving their aim, they should still be offered if the burdens and/or risks are correspondingly low. Those which carry only a small chance of significant prolongation of life should also be offered providing their burdens and risks are not excessive. All treatments considered *obligatory* or *optional* should be discussed with the patient and then provided if the adequately informed patient wishes to undertake them.

It follows from this discussion that burdens and risks always have to be considered in relation to the likelihood and degree of benefit. This is a difficult professional judgement. Such complex and onerous value judgements are part of professional life in palliative care. The responsibility for them cannot be avoided or passed entirely to the patient.

8.4.2   *What morally justifiable criteria should be used to decide what life-prolonging and life-sustaining treatments should be given to non-autonomous patients?*

Whether or not to try to prolong or sustain the life of a non-autonomous patient, whose former wishes are not known, is one of the areas of greatest controversy in health care at present. The moral problems are only slightly less acute in the field of palliative care where we know that the patient is by definition suffering from a terminal illness and so will ultimately die whatever we do.

Much discussion in health care ethics tends to emphasize the importance of respect for autonomy since the Western liberal tradition has seen the value of a person as deriving from their autonomy. How then should the non-autonomous be treated? It must first be remembered that human beings have feelings and sentience as well as reason. Even if a person is no longer mentally competent there is still a duty to minimize suffering and distress. This duty follows from the principle of beneficence. Secondly, the non-autonomous were once autonomous and as such were part of relationships and of a wider community. There is a duty on the part of relatives and the professionals of the community to care for the non-autonomous as still part of that community, even if a fading part. As the poet Shelley puts it:

> *Music, when soft voices die,*
> *Vibrates in the memory;*
> *Odours, when sweet violets sicken*
> *Live within the sense they quicken.*
> *Rose leaves, when the rose is dead,*
> *Are heap'd for the beloved's bed;*
> *And so thy thoughts, when thou art gone,*
> *Love itself shall slumber on.*

To put the point ethically rather than poetically, the duty to care 'until death do us part' follows from the concept of a community.

Many staff who have chosen to work in the field of palliative care have deep religious convictions that all human beings are of value because of their relationship to God. Others without such convictions simply regard all human beings as precious, and will strive to attain as much pleasure, contentment, and comfort for the confused or drowsy patient as possible, whilst caring meticulously for those who are unconscious, just because they are human beings.

In palliative care we deal every day with non-autonomous patients. Almost all patients will have a period of diminished consciousness just before death, and this may extend to several days in many cases. In this situation, a return to an autonomous condition is not usually expected. In contrast, other patients with cerebral tumours, or dementia or mental illness such as schizophrenia coexisting with their terminal illness are non-autonomous for a longer period before death. Yet another group of patients will have temporary loss of autonomy due to biochemical disorders such as hypercalcaemia or renal failure, or they may be excessively sedated for a period as a side-effect of drug administration, or they may simply undergo a period of disorientation if their grip on reality is already fragile. How should patients in these three groups be treated, and why?

The first group of patients, those who have diminished consciousness as a preterminal event, are obviously irreversibly dying, and attempts to prolong life, even if successful, would only prolong dying, which could not be considered a benefit to the patient and is generally considered a harm. Thus mechanical ventilation, renal dialysis, or the insertion of ureteric stents would all be inappropriate at this juncture. In contrast, basic existing life-sustaining treatment, such as insulin for diabetes, would be continued. Steroids should be continued for patients with cerebral tumours where headaches have been a problem and if it is thought that withdrawal of steroids would cause them to increase or recur. If headaches have not been a problem, some carers are happy to stop steroids, on the grounds that they are no longer providing benefit by improving quality of life and have proved physiologically futile because the patient has deteriorated on them. On the other hand, abrupt withdrawal could lead to adrenal failure, which presumably could be unpleasant or might hasten death. Thus opinion is divided on whether steroids should be continued in this situation. Unless the likelihood, consequences, and possible unpleasant symptoms of adrenal failure become better known, there is not likely to be a resolution of this dilemma.

Patients in the other two groups, who are temporarily or permanently confused, demented, or severely mentally ill so that they are incompetent, are not imminently dying. If there is no available advance directive the same lines of reasoning about treatment can be used as those described for autonomous patients. Information about the patient's values and priorities gained from relatives may help health professionals to judge what is in the patient's best interests or total good.

Thus treatments which are very unlikely to achieve their physiological aim, or which entail excessive burdens and/or risks in comparison to their benefits, or which will not further the patient's medical good, or for which resources are not available ought not to be provided. They should be withdrawn or withheld.

We would regard such treatments as those which it is *obligatory not to provide*.

In contrast, treatments for which the burdens and risks do not overwhelmingly outweigh the benefits in terms of the patient's medical good should be regarded as *optional* and considered on their merits in the particular case, and those expected to yield good or moderate benefit with minimal risks and burdens would be regarded as *obligatory to provide*.

Optional treatments for incompetent patients would include such treatments as steroids and radiotherapy for cerebral tumours, tracheostomy for progressive and incurable neck tumours, gastrostomies for incurable obstructive or neurological lesions preventing swallowing, intravenous hydration for patients with intestinal obstruction, antibiotics for those with pneumonia, palliative chemotherapy, bisphosphonates for hypercalcaemia, blood transfusion for anaemia due to incurable marrow insufficiency, and so on. In all these cases the decision to treat or not to treat rests on a benefits to burdens/risks calculus and consideration of the patient's overall medical good in terms of the disease course. Benefits in this context are increased length of a life which it is thought is of some value to the patient, plus any additional benefits of increased comfort.

Professional decisions of this nature are necessarily difficult because they all involve complex value judgements, and also because the benefits and sometimes the burdens and risks of treatment may not be well known. This latter problem arises particularly in issues surrounding artificial hydration when the patient is in a semiconscious or unconscious condition from which it is felt recovery is unlikely. At present we simply do not know whether these patients are distressed by thirst or not, we do not know how great the risk of fluid overload is, or whether poor or absent fluid intake significantly alters the course of the disease, or to what extent such patients might find the treatment of subcutaneous hydration itself burdensome. In the presence of all these uncertainties it is not possible to make a judgement about whether hydration in this circumstance is morally obligatory or optional. Indeed it is possible that future research results may indicate that it is obligatory *not* to provide it (for instance if it proves likely to cause distress and/or fluid overload with little or no benefit to the patient or if it simply prolongs dying).

Until such research (which is fraught with practical and ethical difficulties) reveals the answers to some of these questions, carers will have to continue doing what they believe to be in accord with the patients' medical good. If there is doubt about the value of benefits in comparison with the burdens and risks of a treatment, then we would consider it best to err on the side of non-treatment in the palliative care setting. Benefits may be very uncertain, but often burdens and risks can be more reliably estimated. In general health care there is a presumption in favour of life-prolonging or life-sustaining treatment, but in the palliative care setting where the patient is suffering from an incurable and progressive disease it seems best to presume in favour of non-treatment. This is to avoid the harm of prolonging dying, especially if the treatment entails anything which could be regarded as an intrusion or indignity.

Moreover, non-autonomous patients are extremely vulnerable, and it seems unjustifiable to inflict on them treatment of doubtful value which a competent patient in the same situation might reasonably refuse.

Examples of obligatory treatments for non-autonomous patients in the palliative care context which have a life-sustaining or life-prolonging effect are simple insulin regimes for insulin-dependent diabetics in order to prevent the adverse effects of hypoglycaemia and severe hyperglycaemia, anti-convulsants to prevent fits, bronchodilators if necessary to prevent distress due to asthma, steroids if required to prevent intractable headaches due to a cerebral tumour, and all nursing care appropriate to facilitate comfort.

Professionals working in the palliative care setting bear a heavy responsibility for treatment decisions regarding non-autonomous patients who are totally dependent on them for appropriate care.

8.5 Treatments to alleviate suffering

The problems which occur in the area of symptom control in palliative care do not arise from any uncertainty about the right-ness or wrongness of trying to relieve those symptoms, but rather from the practical and moral difficulties of balancing the benefits, burdens, and risks of treatment. Moreover, usually the moral dilemmas of symptom control relate only to the patient's interests, but occasionally the interests of relatives, and other patients, seem morally relevant and then very difficult moral problems have to be solved.

As with life-prolonging treatments, the moral problems of symptom control for autonomous patients differ in many respects from those relating to the care of non-autonomous patients.

8.5.1   *Moral problems of symptom control in autonomous patients*

Professional carers should select and offer treatments which carry a good or reasonable hope of alleviating distress without entailing excessive burdens and/or risks and which accord with the patient's medical good. Even if the treatment carries a relatively low chance of relieving the symptom it may still be appropriate to offer it if associated burdens and risks are correspondingly low. Once again, it is the balance of benefits versus burdens and risks which is important in selecting treatment. This value judgement, which is often difficult and complex, is inescapable in palliative care.

It follows from our concepts of professional responsibility to benefit and not to harm the patient that treatments which are likely to be futile, or whose harms and risks greatly outweigh their benefits, are not offered. Resource constraints may also decrease the range of treatments available. The extent to which patients want to participate in decision making varies.

Patients who want full participation in decision making
Patients who want full participation in decision making then choose from the treatment options offered, with the benefit of advice from the carers. Together they reach a conclusion regarding the best option in the patient's particular situation. This involves consideration of the patient's wishes and priorities. For instance, patients with bone pain may have different priorities and goals. Some want mobility and will put up with some pain on movement rather than be at all sedated; others are less keen to move about and would rather have complete pain control, even at the cost of less mobility due to some sedation.

Similarly, such patients should be told if a treatment given primarily for symptom control is also likely to influence the length of their life in either direction because this factor is often important in their decision regarding the treatment. Some patients want their life prolonged, but others do not, either because it is of poor quality or little value to them at the present time, or because they consider that it will be of poor quality or little value to them in the future. For example, the symptoms of a chest infection occurring in the very frail can be alleviated by antibiotics which cure the infection but may well also prolong life. Patients who do not want this may prefer to opt for other methods of symptom control such as cough suppressants or sedatives. Antibiotics would be offered if they carried a good chance of benefit with relatively low burdens and risks, but patients who wish to be fully involved in decision making might decline them.

We have already discussed the clinical situation in which the autonomous patient requests symptom control which they know may have a foreseen effect of shortening life (see Chapter 5). Such patients may no longer consider death a harm, or may consider it to be only a minor harm in comparison with pain and other forms of distress. Any effects of a treatment which may hasten death are then of less importance to them than the goal of alleviating distress. Carers are then faced with the difficult judgement of whether the possible shortening of life in the situation is justified by the benefits the treatment will confer. Usually in this situation both carers and patients agree that the balance of benefits over harms justifies the treatment requested. Those who consider that it is never permissible to shorten life intentionally will use the doctrine of double effect (see Chapter 5) but many others feel that the balance of benefits to burdens in this clinical situation is sufficient justification. Sometimes this clinical judgement is difficult. For example, patients who have become quadriplegic or paraplegic due to cord compression resulting from malignancy have a poor prognosis but may not be imminently dying, and they may occasionally request sedation to escape from the severe mental shock and distress of their present condition and future prospects. Carers then have to justify the effects of such sedation, including effects which may hasten death. Full discussion between the patient and the team, with explanations to the family, is essential in this difficult situation.

Patients who do not want full participation in decision making
Some patients do want wish to choose from a range of options and prefer to describe their own priorities and then ask the professional to recommend the treatment which is considered most appropriate in their case. This course of action represents a conscious choice to trust the professional's knowledge and dedication to the patient's good. Many tired or frightened patients who do not want a detailed

discussion of options prefer to take this course, and their decision to do so should be respected.

8.5.2 Moral problems of symptom control in non-autonomous patients

As in the preceding discussion on life-prolonging treatments, non-autonomous patients can be considered in two groups for the purposes of discussion; those who are actually dying and those who are not imminently dying but are confused or mentally ill.

Physical comfort and relief of psychological distress are the priorities of care for those who are dying. As we have said, treatment essential for comfort is not withheld even if it may have a secondary effect of shortening life. In contrast, it might be said that some treatments to alleviate symptoms may have a significant effect in prolonging dying, and this may constitute a harm which then has to be weighed against the benefits of such treatment. Measures such as antibiotics for what is considered to be a terminal chest infection, and intravenous or subcutaneous hydration in a dying patient, are often withheld partly because the possible (though often unlikely) benefit of alleviating symptoms is outweighed by the harm of prolonging dying. Instead other methods of symptom control are used, which are believed to be effective without entailing a risk of prolonging dying.

Patients who are not imminently dying but who are confused and disorientated, demented, or mentally ill, either as a consequence of or in addition to their terminal illness, are often quite capable of making a range of decisions or of indicating preferences. When a treatment decision arises which it is thought the patient may comprehend, every reasonable attempt should be made to enable the patient to participate in the decision. Staff will endeavour to explain the clinical situation so as to enable the patient to indicate a choice or preference. If this fails, either because the patient cannot comprehend the information, or retain it long enough for consideration, or reach a conclusion by the use of reason, then the patient is incompetent to make the decision. If a patient is completely dysphasic it may not be possible to ascertain if the patient is competent, and it is often impossible for any conclusion to be communicated to the carers. For practical purposes such a patient is incompetent to make a decision.

We have said that the responsibility of carers towards patients who are incompetent is to provide treatment following a benefits to burdens/risks calculus. However, the final assessment of the magnitude of benefits and harms is dependent on the patient's attitude towards them. Substantially non-autonomous patients are unable to carry out such assessments, and so carers are limited in their ability to formulate the benefits to burdens/risks calculus in this situation. They have then to rely on experience gained with other patients, on their knowledge of this particular patient gained through personal contact, and on information about the patient's values and priorities gained from friends and relatives. Decisions made in this way are often very difficult, and the carers' judgement about which treatment is actually best for the patient is more likely to prove wrong. Therefore, frequent review of treatments and willingness to change them are morally required. For example, it is often difficult to assess whether the apparatus used for some treatments, such as syringe drivers or intravenous infusions, will cause distress which is disproportionate to the benefit of the treatment. Sometimes the best course of action is to try the treatment and be ready to discontinue it if it causes excessive distress.

A difficult moral question arises, and has to be considered in the light (or perhaps the darkness) of all these uncertainties—is it ever morally justifiable to force a treatment on an unwilling patient who is not competent to make the decision but who is distressed by a symptom? We consider that occasionally it is, and the commonest situation in palliative care where this practice is morally justified is the alleviation of psychological distress or pain in a confused, agitated, and perhaps paranoid patient. If the reassurance of calm human contact and familiar company fails, and physical causes have been excluded or treated, yet the patient is distressed but refuses oral medication, then it is appropriate and justifiable to give a sedative by injection to relieve distress, restore dignity, and enable analgesia to be given if required. The benefits of this course of action often outweigh the harm of giving an injection to an unwilling patient.

8.6 The role of relatives

The moral dilemmas of palliative care usually relate only to the patient's best interests, but sometimes the interests of relatives are relevant. We have discussed possible conflicts of interest in Chapters 3 and 5, where we stressed that priority must be given to the patient's interests. However, where relatives are actively involved in the care of the patient, their ability and/or willingness to participate in care is highly relevant. This is discussed further in Chapter 9 on other management decisions.

Autonomous patients will make decisions about treatment in a discussion partnership with the professional carers. Such patients will take the relatives' views and interests into account. The professionals' responsibility is to act in accordance with the patient's good. The relatives' interests should not influence the professional carers' decision.

This may seem hard or even unjust, but if the financial or other interests of relatives were permitted to influence the professionals' decisions directly in these matters, then the welfare of all patients in this situation would be compromised. For example, professionals should not be influenced against providing life-prolonging treatment because the relatives either do not want to meet nursing home costs, or do not feel willing or able to undertake the patient's care. Carers should not be persuaded by the relatives' interests to advise the patient against antibiotics for pneumonia or other life-prolonging or life-sustaining treatments. Decisions should be made in the patient's interests, not those of the relatives. Put crudely, this means that we must not be influenced to 'let patients die' because life would be easier for those around them if they were dead.

Western societies are facing the upwardly spiralling costs of caring for an increasingly elderly and dependent population. We have said that if a treatment is available in terms of resources, then resource considerations should not influence decisions regarding its use for a particular patient. Unfortunately, in a climate of relative lack of health care resources it would be easy for carers to use the interests of relatives as an additional reason to withhold or withdraw life-prolonging or life-sustaining measures. It is partly because of this climate of competition for resources that the relatives' interests cannot be allowed to influence decisions about life-prolonging treatment. Of course it could be argued, on the other hand, that society's interests influence life-prolonging treatment via resource constraints, so it is inconsistent to say that relatives' financial interests should not also be considered. Increasingly, the resource consequences for continuing care are being passed on to relatives who must have some say in how their resources are used.

Similarly, the relatives' interests should not influence professionals to initiate or continue life-prolonging or life-sustaining treatment if it is considered that such treatment is not in the patient's best interests. Palliative care specialists sometimes say that 'the family is the unit of care.' This statement should not be taken to mean that the relatives' interests should override those of the patient, whether the latter is autonomous or not.

Non-autonomous patients usually have relatives or close friends who know them well enough to be able to inform professionals of the patient's values and preferences. They may be asked to state what they think the patient would have wanted in the circumstances. This is called a substitute judgement. Many relatives feel unwilling to take this responsibility, or are unable to do so because they never discussed with the patient the circumstances which have actually arisen. Nevertheless they are able to provide valuable insights into the patient's values and priorities, and can help the professional carers to plan and provide treatment in accordance with the patient's medical good and total good in so far as the latter can be surmised. We have already discussed these issues in another context (Chapter 3, pp. 58–65).

In some circumstances the interests of the non-autonomous patient seem inextricably mixed with those of relatives who are providing care, and in this situation we have said that the interests of the relatives are a legitimate and essential consideration. For example, dexamethasone is often used for patients with cerebral tumours in order to maintain neurological function, especially speech and movement, and to alleviate headaches. Unfortunately, it can cause hyperactivity which results in exhaustion on behalf of the relative caring for the patient who wishes to be at home. Does one then reduce the dexamethasone, which entails a risk of deterioration in neurological function and onset of headaches, in order to spare the relative, or not? This complex decision can be resolved only by application of the benefits to burdens/risks calculus for the patient. One solution is to provide regular day centre or respite care, and to sedate the patient at night, in order to enable the benefits of the dexamethasone to be gained whilst at the same time enabling the relative to cope at home, which is where the patient wishes to be.

Ultimately, the members of the professional team are responsible for their decisions regarding treatment for the non-autonomous patient. Responsibility for those difficult treatment choices cannot be passed to the relatives, but must remain with those who either provide or withhold the treatment. Relatives have a responsibility to inform the carers about the patient's known wishes, values, and preferences, but they do not have and cannot assume responsibility for the treatment decisions made as a result of that information.

8.7 Conflicts of interest between patients

In an in-patient unit or day centre, conflicts of interest between patients themselves always pose difficult moral dilemmas, because the carers have moral responsibilities to all the patients. For example, if dying patients make an expiratory noise arising from the larynx, or resulting from secretions in the throat, other patients (and indeed relatives) may be distressed. In contrast, the dying and unconscious patient is very unlikely to be distressed. Usually in this situation the dying patient will be given muscle relaxants such as diazepam to try to reduce grunting, and hyoscine to reduce secretions, but if these medications fail to reduce sounds which distress other patients, the dying patient is often moved to a single room. The medication and the possible move are justified because they do not harm the dying patient, and benefit the others. It is worth noting that sometimes other patients do not want the dying patient moved for their sake—great altruism is seen in groups of terminally ill people cared for together.

Confused, demented, or mentally ill patients, especially those whose behaviour is threatening if not actually violent, can cause considerable distress to those around them, who may be so incapacitated by their illness that they cannot move away. In this situation it seems morally justifiable to sedate the confused patient as much as is necessary to protect others from distress, and those who are threatening or actually violent should be moved to a suitable unit in cooperation with the psychiatric service. Even though it may be in the interests of the confused patient to remain in a specialist palliative care unit, harm to other patients cannot be justified. In a more common example, we accept that confused patients who keep others awake at night should be sedated, whether they like it or not!

8.8   Reassessment of treatment decisions

It is important that professional carers, patients, and relatives understand that treatment decisions made at a particular time and in particular circumstances are valid only at that time and in those circumstances. Treatment decisions need to be reviewed regularly, at least as often as significant changes in the patient's condition or wishes occur or if other circumstances affecting their care change. No treatment decision is written in tablets of stone.

Moreover, since there are so many uncertainties in the factors considered when palliative care decisions are made, many decisions will turn out with hindsight not to have given the optimum result, and the treatments will need to be changed or modified.

In the chapter on clinical decision making we explained that it is philosophically unsound and also unhelpful in clinical practice to make a moral distinction between withholding and withdrawing treatment, even if that treatment is sustaining or prolonging life. Such a treatment should be commenced if indicated, and withdrawn if it is unhelpful or harmful or if the patient's circumstances change and it is no longer indicated. It is not morally defensible to avoid commencing a treatment which is indicated because of reluctance to discontinue it in the future when it is no longer indicated.

8.9   Autonomous to non-autonomous conditions

In palliative care, professionals can often foresee likely events in the course of the illness which may render the patient incompetent to participate further in necessary treatment decisions. Wherever possible, without causing excessive trauma to the patient, it is good practice to attempt to discuss with patients what treatment they would want if these events took place and they became incompetent to participate in decisions. At the same time we must acknowledge that patients may not want to try to foresee future illness scenarios, and it is easy to traumatize such patients by pursuing discussions about future events in order to make future decision making easier. Such traumatization of patients is surely not justified by the argument that it is more likely that health care professionals will be aware of the patient's previously stated wishes when difficult decisions have to be made.

Discussion with patients about possible future events during the course of the illness gives the carers the advantage of knowing what those patients thought they would want and not want in terms of treatment, and the patients' wishes can be respected. The other considerable advantage is that of enabling patients to be as fully informed as possible about those events. This enables them to consider their wishes carefully in the light of a full understanding of their likely future circumstances, and they can give instructions as to what treatment they might want. It is obviously important to record such instructions carefully in the patient's notes, and to discuss them with other colleagues likely to be involved. Some patients may want to make a formal advance directive, but more often they simply want to make their wishes known to those responsible for their treatment, leaving some discretion as to how to interpret those wishes in the circumstances which do eventually arise.

8.10   Advance statements and proxy decision makers

Advance statements and the role of proxy decision makers are best considered separately because their use in clinical decisions leads to different moral problems.

8.10.1   *Advance statements*

Advance statements (sometimes called living wills) are written or oral statements which people make whilst mentally competent in order to influence treatment decisions which arise when they are no longer competent to make those decisions. The statements come into force only after the onset of mental incompetence (also referred to as mental incapacity). The requirements for competence or capacity to make a treatment decision are discussed in detail in Chapter 9; it is important to note that in order to be competent to make a decision the patient must be adequately informed and able to understand and to retain the information relevant to the decision, and to assess it and arrive at a free choice. Advance statements are intended for use when the patient lacks competence to make the decision. They are always superseded by a decision made by a patient who is competent. The

British Medical Association (BMA) issued a code of practice (British Medical Association, 1995) regarding advance statements in order to clarify their use in clinical decision making.

Just as patients vary in the amount of involvement that they want in clinical decision making when competent, so they also vary in the amount of influence that they wish to exert, via an advance statement, over decisions which arise when they are no longer competent. Thus, just as they should be able to choose the nature and extent of their involvement in decisions when competent, so they should also be free to choose the nature of the advance statement they wish to make, and the extent to which it relates to specific treatments or clinical states. In recognizing this the BMA drew attention to the fact that an advance statement can take various forms:

- 'A statement of the general beliefs and aspects of life which an individual values. This provides a summary of individual responses to a list of questions about their past and present wishes and future desires. It makes no specific request or refusal but attempts to give a biographical portrait of the individual as an aid to deciding what he or she would want.'
- 'A requesting statement reflecting an individual's aspirations and preferences. This can help professionals identify how the person would like to be treated without binding them to that course of action, if it conflicts with professional judgement.'
- 'A clear instruction refusing some or all medical procedures (advance directive). Made by a competent adult, this does, in certain circumstances, have legal force.'
- 'A statement which, rather than refusing any particular treatment, specifies a degree of irreversible deterioration (such as a diagnosis of persistent vegetative state) after which no life-sustaining treatment should be given. For adults, this again can have legal force.'
- 'A statement which names another person who should be consulted at the time a decision has to be made. The views expressed by that named person should reflect what the patient would want. This can supplement and clarify the intended scope of a written statement but the named person's views are presently not legally binding in England and Wales. In Scotland, the powers of a tutor dative may cover such eventualities.'

- 'A combination of the above, including requests, refusals and the nomination of a representative. Those sections expressing clear refusal may have legal force in the case of adult patients.'

This description of the many ways in which an advance statement may be made emphasizes to both patients and professional carers that the choice of exactly what an advance statement comprises is a matter of individual patient preference. Some patients may simply want to give information about their values and priorities so as to help professionals to assess their 'total good'; for example, they might state that they have always valued physical independence and mental clarity and the ability to relate to their family. Others may want to indicate a preference for, or refusal of, certain forms of treatment in certain circumstances; for example, they might want to decline renal dialysis if terminally ill or mentally incapacitated. Others may wish to request or refuse life-sustaining treatment after some degree of irreversible deterioration; for example, they might want to refuse life-prolonging treatment if they were irreversibly mentally incapacitated or unconscious. The moral problems of choosing friends or relatives to act as proxy decision makers are discussed later.

An obvious drawback of making an advance statement relating to specific treatments or circumstances is that people may not know beforehand how they will feel when in a situation which they have never experienced, yet despite this many people quite understandably wish to influence decisions regarding life-prolonging or life-sustaining treatment on the basis of what they think their wishes would be.

Another obvious difficulty for those making advance statements relating to specific treatments or clinical circumstances is that they cannot know in advance exactly what circumstances are going to arise, and so it is difficult to give instructions which are obviously applicable to the circumstances which do arise. For example, if someone wants to decline artificial nutrition and hydration if he is in the persistent vegetative state, then that advance statement applies only to the circumstance of being in that state, and not to any other condition giving rise to unconsciousness. It is statistically very unlikely that the outcome of an illness or accident might be the persistent vegetative state. Thus a very specific directive is less likely to be applicable to the circumstances which later occur. On the other hand, a very non-specific directive may be difficult to interpret because it may not be clear whether it does apply in the situation which has arisen. For example, if an advance statement states that the patient does not want life-prolonging measures if he is irreversibly confused, then was that directive intended to refuse insulin if the patient is a diabetic, and does it apply if the confusion is only mild and the patient not distressed? Therefore, making statements which will clearly apply to the actual circumstances which will later arise necessitates the careful description of the nature and range of possible circumstances and treatments which the patient wishes to consider in the statement.

In palliative care the diagnosis and likely course of the illness is known, and so future events can to some extent be anticipated, and the future treatment options can likewise often be anticipated. Patients who wish to make advance statements relating to future specific treatments and clinical circumstances will need to be informed about those events and treatments in order to be competent to make such a statement. In the context of palliative care such discussions will necessarily involve a dialogue about the various ways of dying of the illness. Not all patients will wish to receive this information, and they may prefer to make a statement about general values and priorities, or to describe in broad terms those clinical conditions in which they would not want their lives artificially prolonged or sustained by medical interventions. Giving information to those who do want to make statements regarding specific treatments in certain circumstances will require great sensitivity.

It is important to note that advance refusals of treatment (for which the BMA reserve the term advance directive) are legally binding if valid and applicable under the circumstances which have arisen. A refusal is valid if made by an adequately informed person who was capable of understanding the nature and consequences of the decision, and was able to retain that information and arrive at a choice free of undue pressure. It is obvious that an advance refusal of treatment may result in the patient's death, or in the survival of the patient in a condition which is substantially worse than could have been achieved if the treatment had been given. The latter consequence may occur if a patient has declined ventilation, and develops a chest infection which is not fatal, but the withholding of ventilation results in hypoxic brain damage leading to survival with long-term disability. Some evidence that the patient appreciated the consequences of refusal is necessary to establish that the refusal is valid. A refusal is applicable if the circumstances which have arisen are those which the patient envisaged when the directive was written, and to which the refusal was intended to apply. When an advance refusal is valid and applicable, it is respected in the same way as the contemporaneous refusal of treatment by a competent person. It can be seen that the judgement of whether an advance refusal is valid and applicable carries major consequences for the patient's future (and incidentally for friends and relatives as well). Such a judgement is of very great practical, as well as legal, importance. It is likely that many professional carers will seek legal advice in order to assess the evidence concerning validity and applicability of refusals of treatment if there is any doubt.

The BMA code of practice 'provides that as a matter of public policy, people should not be able to refuse basic care in advance or instruct others to refuse it on their behalf.' Basic care means those medical treatments and nursing measures essential to provide comfort and alleviate pain or distress. It includes provision of warmth, shelter, hygiene measures, and management of distressing symptoms such as pain and breathlessness, and provision of oral food and fluids (but not artificial feeding by nasogastric tube, gastrostomy, or parenteral routes, which may all be declined via an advance statement).

It seems reasonable to suggest that professionals involved in palliative care should show willingness to discuss the likely future course of the illness with patients, and should encourage those who show a desire to influence their future management when incompetent to make an advance statement, either written or oral. It is important to stress to patients that the sort of statement made is a matter of individual choice. It is also important that patients understand that any advance statement can be changed or revoked by the competent patient at any time, either orally or in writing.

The BMA code of practice relating to advance statements solves some moral problems, in that it stresses patient choice in making the statement, and makes clear that basic care cannot be refused, and that emergency treatment should not be withheld whilst an advance statement is found or interpreted. It states that statements requesting a certain treatment cannot legally bind carers to initiate that treatment if in their professional judgement it is inappropriate. This might be because it is physiologically futile, not in accord with

the patient's medical good, or not available due to resource constraints. The code states clearly the requirements for capacity to
make a decision, and therefore capacity to make an advance statement relating to a specific decision, and it also makes clear the
legally binding nature of a valid and applicable advance refusal of
treatment. However, some moral problems remain. It may be very
difficult to establish in some cases whether an advance refusal is
valid and applicable. In addition, all ambiguities implied in the use
of some terms cannot be eliminated. For example, the scope of what
is considered life-sustaining treatment is uncertain—is insulin such a
treatment, and if so should it be stopped if a patient refuses all life-
sustaining treatment in certain circumstances, or is insulin essential
for patient comfort, and therefore part of basic care? Similarly, it
may be difficult to decide what constitutes a terminal illness, or at
what point a condition is irreversible. When these difficulties arise
it is likely that legal advice will be sought, but it also appears that
the costs of such advice will be met out of the budget for patient
care. Thus the use of advance statements could consume considerable human and financial resources from the total available for
health care.

These examples serve to illustrate that giving information and
advice to patients making advance statements, and interpreting those
statements whilst making decisions for incompetent patients, are
difficult and complex tasks which ultimately are the responsibility of
health care professionals. Advance statements should assist health
care professionals to make decisions for incompetent patients that
will further the total good (legally termed 'best interests') of those
patients, but achieving this goal will require practical wisdom as
well as all the professional skills described in this chapter and in
Chapter 5 on clinical decision making.

8.10.2 Proxy decision makers

Proxy decision makers are people appointed by patients when
competent in order to make treatment choices on behalf of the
patient when incompetent. At present, in the United Kingdom, the
proxy has no legal authority to consent to or refuse treatment on
behalf of the patient. However, the role of the proxy is to participate
in discussion of treatment options on behalf of the patient, if asked
to do so as described in the advance statement.

If the proxy has knowledge of the treatment the patient would have chosen in the circumstances in question, based on previous discussions about those circumstances, then the proxy is able to indicate what the patient would have wanted in those circumstances.

If no such discussion took place, the proxy has to recommend the management which he or she considers the patient would have wished on the basis of close knowledge of the patient's values and preferences. In this situation the proxy has to interpret the patient's previous statements about values and priorities in the light of the current circumstances and then make a judgement of what the patient would have wanted. If unable or unwilling to do this the proxy may make a statement of what he or she feels is in the patients best interests, based on knowledge of the patient.

In fact, spouses and other close family members are often used as proxy decision makers for incompetent patients as described earlier, even though they were not officially appointed as such by the patient. One of the major difficulties is that both official and unofficial proxy decision makers are usually so close to the patient that they may have personal interests at stake in the patient's management, and this may influence their opinions concerning management. They may also be unwilling to shoulder the responsibility of influencing the treatment of the patient, feeling that whatever they say they may subsequently feel guilty about their part in bringing about the eventual outcome.

8.11 Conclusions

1. Treatment options are selected by carers on the basis of the benefits to burdens/risks calculus. They are then offered to autonomous patients, or considered by carers and relatives on behalf of non-autonomous patients.
2. Treatments should not be given if they are physiologically futile, or if their associated burdens and risks greatly outweigh their benefits.
3. Autonomous patients should choose the extent to which they wish to participate in decisions about these treatments; if they wish to be fully involved they must be adequately informed. This means that they need to know the likely future course of

the illness with and without treatment, as well as the burdens, risks, and possible benefits of treatment.

4. Non-autonomous patients are unable to participate in deriving the balance of benefits to burdens and risks in the particular situation. Information from relatives about the patient's wishes, values, and priorities is very important in establishing the magnitude and significance of the benefits and harms for the particular patient.

5. The rightness or wrongness of life-prolonging and life-sustaining treatments in palliative care depends on the particular clinical circumstances in which they are considered.

6. Since the outcome of treatments is always uncertain because of the unpredictability of the disease course and the uncertainties of the benefits to burdens/risks calculus, treatments should be reviewed regularly and carers should always remain willing to modify treatment accordingly.

7. Carers should not intend to cause overall harm to patients in the interests of relatives, but it is sometimes morally justifiable to compromise the good of one patient in the interests of others.

8. Advance statements will be difficult to write and may prove difficult to interpret. The patient's wishes should be respected with regard to valid and applicable refusals of treatment, but advance statements cannot bind carers to provide treatment which they feel is clinically inappropriate.

9

Other management decisions

I am a very foolish fond old man.
Fourscore and upward, not an hour more nor less;
And, to deal plainly, I fear I am not in my perfect mind.
Shakespeare, *King Lear* (1606)

9.1 Problems of autonomy and competence

In the preceding chapters we have discussed treatment decisions in terms of the concept of autonomy, and we have recognized that autonomy is a spectrum phenomenon. One element in the broad concept of autonomy is that concerned specifically with our ability to make decisions. This element is often called 'competence' or 'capacity', and we shall use this conceptual derivative of autonomy to address the specific problem of patient decision making.

Competence, like autonomy, is a spectrum phenomenon. No patient has complete and perfect understanding of the illness and of all the available treatments and their associated benefits, burdens, and risks. Many patients have a limited ability to believe the information given, especially if shocked by 'bad news', and can have difficulty evaluating the information in the context of their own lives. They may also be unduly influenced by relatives or professionals, so that their decision may not be substantially free and voluntary. Competence also entails the ability to make a rational decision. Analysis of what it means to 'reach a rational conclusion' in decision-making is problematic. We shall simply accept that a rational decision is one made on the basis of reasoning, even if that reasoning is imperfect, or if the patient chooses a course of action which is not that which appears best to the average person.

The important practical issue is whether the patient is *adequately competent* to make the decision in question, and this assessment of competence can be very difficult in the clinical situation, giving rise to serious moral problems. Patients are judged competent to make a decision if they are:

1. informed of the facts and probabilities
2. able to understand and believe the facts and probabilities
3. able to make a voluntary choice (absence of coercion)
4. able to make a reasoned choice
5. able to communicate that choice.

Moral problems regarding judgements about competence arise particularly when a patient refuses treatment, or with regard to decisions about place of care. If a patient requests treatment and it is uncertain whether he or she is competent to do so, the treatment does not have to be given if the professional team consider that it is not in the patient's interests. In this case the professionals are entitled to override the patient's request. However, it is much more difficult to override a refusal of treatment—this can be done only if it can be shown that the patient is definitely not competent to make the decision. The burden of proof lies with the carers.

Similarly, it is difficult to override a patient's wish to remain at home—patients can be removed from home against their will only if they are shown to be incompetent to make a decision regarding place of care, and the burden of proof once again lies with the carers. In contrast, patients can be refused entry to certain places of institutional care for reasons of medical or nursing need or resource constraints. Clinical examples illustrate these problems and demonstrate that there are no rules which appear to give satisfactory outcomes in all cases.

Some patients have irrational fears, including fears of interventions such as drips or needles, operations or anaesthetics. Suppose a patient who has been on large doses of oral opiates for pain control then becomes unable to take the medication orally. The best (and for the sake of the argument the only) way to give adequate analgesia is then via a subcutaneous syringe-driver or injections, both of which involve needles. Such a patient may refuse the analgesia because of an irrational fear of needles. Whilst it can be argued that this patient's mind is dominated by this irrational fear, and that the patient is too weak-willed to be able to exercise choice, in fact it is not possible to overrule the patient and give parenteral analgesia unless he or she becomes overtly confused or virtually unconscious. The patient is likely to acknowledge that his fears are irrational, but ultimately the choice to refuse treatment has to be accepted; it is the patient's right to refuse consent. The fact that others consider the decision to be against the patient's best interests, and may consider the reasons implausible, is not relevant. In this situation the patient is competent and the decision must be respected. In practice, treatment alternatives and compromises will be offered, such as sedation to lessen the fear, application of potent anaesthetic creams at the cannula site, and so on, and it is always hoped that the irrational fear may be overcome so that treatment which the patient acknowledges to be beneficial and offers the best outcome can be given.

More serious irrational fears and false beliefs sometimes cost patients their lives. For example, a young woman with an irrational fear that mastectomy or lumpectomy would cause her breast cancer to spread declined the operation and developed a massive fungating local breast cancer and later died. She might have been cured by surgery when she had presented in the early stages of the illness. Her decision was based on reasoning, but that reasoning was based on a false belief and irrational fear of the operation. Despite these factors her refusal to consent to what was possibly curative treatment had to be accepted even though it was acknowledged that she would die of the cancer. She believed (it may be considered irrationally) that she could combat and overcome the illness by determination.

Some patients have an overwhelming fear of death which may appear irrational, and so will demand any treatment which offers a chance, however small, to put off death. For example, some patients would request a chemotherapy regime associated with only a 2 per cent chance of prolonging life for only a few months, even though there is a 98 per cent chance that the regime will yield only harms and risks and no benefit. Such treatment is sometimes given to them, even though it could be argued that they are driven by this intense fear, and even though they may acknowledge that their decision is not logically the best. The treatment is given out of respect for their autonomy even though it could be argued that their autonomy is significantly diminished, and it is acknowledged that the treatment is likely to cause a balance of harm over good.

In these examples the fact that the patient's decision is based on reasoning is considered sufficient to meet the 'rationality' requirement of competence for making the decision. This is so even though the reasons given might be considered invalid by others, and even though the reasoning process may be imperfect, and even though the patient may admit that the decision made is not in accord with the best outcome as indicated by deliberations.

Thus patients' refusals of treatment, even if based on irrational fears or false beliefs, tend to be accepted unless that patient is obviously totally confused, seriously deluded, or unconscious. This is done in order to support and observe the principle of respect for autonomy, even if diminished, and because we take the view that rationality relating to competence means 'based on reasoning', and does not require that the reasons be valid or that the reasoning process be perfect.

This interpretation and practical application of the principle of respect for autonomy has some unfortunate consequences in terms of patients' suffering and sometimes death, but it is considered that it would be more harmful in general to allow carers to override refusals of treatment, and so the 'costs' of refusals based on irrational fears and false beliefs are accepted. Similarly respect for autonomy makes carers reluctant to refuse to provide life-prolonging or life-sustaining treatments even when their attendant risks and burdens are extremely high. However, whilst health care professionals are bound not to override refusal of treatment by competent patients, they are not bound to acquiesce to requests for treatment which in their view is overwhelmingly likely to cause overall harm rather than benefit.

Patients in the palliative care setting are presumed adequately autonomous and competent to make a decision until proved otherwise. The patient's decision is likely to be respected even though its consequences are bad for the patient and others, and even though the patient's capacity to understand and retain the necessary information and make a truly voluntary and rational decision is in doubt.

In the clinical situation this is done for two reasons; firstly out of respect for whatever autonomy the patient has, and secondly because professional carers and relatives naturally want to give terminally ill patients what they want, however irrational and contrary to the patient's interests it may seem. These two reasons are quite distinct. Whilst we would agree that it is desirable to respect whatever autonomy patients do have, and wherever possible to encourage and enable patients to make those decisions which they are competent to make, we do not consider that professional carers should do whatever the patient wants just because the patient wants it. Some examples help to illustrate this point.

If a terminally ill patient feels lethargic, is not motivated to be independent, but is not imminently dying, then members of a specialist palliative care team will encourage the patient to change position, sit out of bed, and be as mobile as possible in order to prevent pressure sores and to maintain some degree of independence. Such patients will be encouraged strongly to get out of bed, and in the in-patient setting it is very difficult for them to refuse. The team members exert their influence in the interests of the patient's medical good and do not easily acquiesce and allow the patient to lie in bed constantly. It is their professional responsibility to act in the patient's best interests. Relatives and non-specialist carers may be inclined to leave the patient in bed day and night, believing that if you are dying the least others can do is grant your requests, whether on balance they seem reasonable or not!

Sometimes it is necessary and justifiable to override the patient's autonomy because the law or professional regulations require it. For example, cot-sides are put up to prevent patients who are undergoing an anaesthetic from falling out of bed, and patients over a certain specified weight are lifted by a hoist rather than two nurses, in order to prevent injury to the nurses' backs.

9.2   Alternative therapy

Many patients who have been told they have an incurable illness seek and pursue alternative therapy in order to try to cure the disease or retard its progress. The efficacy of such therapies is often regarded as unproven because they have not been subjected to rigorous clinical trials. Nevertheless it is acknowledged that they may be effective in retarding the disease, that they probably have a useful placebo effect, and that many patients feel psychologically better as a result of the treatments (such as relaxation therapy) and because they feel they are doing something to help themselves. It is generally believed that alternative therapies have very few side-effects or risks, although they may be quite burdensome to the patient.

Moral problems arise for orthodox professionals whom patients may ask about alternative therapies. Doctors in particular may find themselves torn between wanting patients to obtain any possible benefit from the treatment but being worried at the same time that unreasonable claims may be made by therapists about the efficacy of the treatment. They may also be concerned that some harmful effects may ensue, especially if patients choose to abandon conventional therapy (which offers no hope of cure) for alternative therapy which they have been told will cure them. It seems that the only justifiable course of action is for the professional to be honest with the patient about the uncertainty of benefit from the alternative therapy, just as honesty about the uncertainty of benefit from many conventional treatments is morally required. It is also appropriate to be honest about the dangers of forgoing conventional treatment, and about any burdens or risks attached to the alternative therapy. For example, large doses of some vitamins are harmful, and some of the diets recommended by homeopathists are burdensome to patients who sometimes find it difficult to maintain their weight on a very unfamiliar and restrictive dietary regime.

Sometimes patients are told that they are improving by those providing complementary or alternative therapy. If this is obviously untrue on the basis of clinical evidence, and the patient seeks the opinion of the doctor or nurse, then an honest opinion should be given as gently as possible even though the patient may be disappointed. This seems the most morally acceptable approach unless it is proved in the future that simple belief in progress and cure will bring about disease regression, symptom relief, or cure.

Truth-telling to patients and relatives can also pose problems with regard to alternative therapy. For example, an elderly man with advanced liver cancer had exhausted all forms of conventional treatment with no response. He was on medication to maintain electrolyte balance which had become deranged as a result of inappropriate ADH secretion. He and his wife and son were keen to pursue homeopathic treatment involving a complex organic vegetable diet, enemas, and vitamins, and to this end they went to a homeopathy treatment centre in South America. Having faith in the treatment offered there, which they were told could be curative, the patient discontinued his medication to maintain electrolyte balance. His condition deteriorated as a result of this and because the diet and enemas compounded the electrolyte problems. He returned home to the United Kingdom very ill indeed, but improved on taking his medication again. His wife asked if the homeopathy regime had been harmful. Should she have been told, as the carers believed, that the omission of his regular medication combined with the homeopathy regime had nearly killed him?

At this time she was trying desperate
vegetable diet which he was rejecting
explain to his wife that he could no lor
did not seem to have been effective a
advanced, and that he could no long
not actually told that their pursuit o
exclusion of conventional therapy had
that this knowledge would cause feel
strongly encouraged him to pursue
respectful of her autonomy, and if so, was withholding the truth
justifiable on the grounds that it might spare her guilt?

If conventional treatment ultimately causes harm to patients who
then ask if this has indeed occurred, it seems that they should be told
honestly that whilst it seemed the best decision at the time the
disease failed to respond and harms of the treatment were incurred.
There does not seem to be a moral justification for misleading
patients with regard to the possible adverse effects of conventional
treatment they have had. Unfortunately, the legal situation with
regard to this sort of query can be very complex, and may lead
medical defence and professional organizations to advise professionals not to admit that patients may have been harmed by
treatment.

Faith healing can occasionally pose problems if patients are told
that they will be made well if only they have enough faith. Unfortunately, they may then feel guilty if they do not improve or are
not cured, because they will attribute this failure to lack of faith.
Carers may feel justified in reassuring such patients that in their
experience others with great faith have not been cured, and that it is
not generally thought that lack of faith causes disease, deterioration,
and death, or that lack of faith impedes any beneficial effect of faith
healing.

9.3 Place of care

In palliative care much emphasis is put on the moral importance of
enabling patients to live and particularly to die in the place of their
choice. We would wish to add that it is respecting the patient's
contemporaneous choice which is important. In other words, if a
patient initially decides he wants to die at home, and then later

s mind and requests hospital or specialist palliative care n his later wish should be respected, and regrets should not pressed that he did not die at home unless the available services d not provided all the care they could. It seems that as people become more ill and require more physical care, and perhaps become increasingly aware of the physical and emotional strains on their family, and perhaps also want the reassurance of the presence of continuous nursing and medical assistance, they tend to ask for admission to in-patient care. This does not represent a failure of care at home and should not be regarded as such unless, as we have said, the domiciliary services available were not correctly used. Resource constraints necessarily mean that continuous professional care cannot be provided at home; to do so would require that other branches of the health care services were unjustly penalized financially because the costs of one-to-one care in the patient's home are so high.

We would therefore begin by saying that the professional team should aim to provide the necessary care where the patient wants to be at the time, but within the constraints of the resources available. The resources available at home include the mental, emotional, and physical energy and ability of relatives and friends as well as the community health care services. Unavoidable limitations of the resources available at home are likely to influence patients' decisions regarding place of care during the illness and at the time of death.

Some of the moral problems surrounding the place of care arise because of a certain asymmetry in the way that the patient's right to be at home is viewed. Patients who are at home and wish to remain there cannot be removed against their wishes unless they are clearly shown to be incompetent to make the decision about place of care. Once incompetent, they will be moved only if to do so will not cause them harm. For instance, ambulance crews will not normally move an imminently dying patient who may not survive the journey to hospital, or whose condition might deteriorate considerably as a result of the journey. In other words, the patient's interests are considered paramount in the question of such a move.

In contrast, it is the case in the United Kingdom that once patients are in institutional care and are physically dependent they can be discharged only if the caring team have made a full assessment of their needs and demonstrated that a care plan is in place to meet those needs, in accordance with the NHS and Community Care Act

(1990). The only alternative open to patients who want to go home is self-discharge. This latter process is necessarily confrontational and entails signing a form which usually states that readmission may be denied. Thus when a patient who needs a 'reasonable' amount of care wants to go home, a full Community Care Assessment is legally required and the patient can be discharged by the team if, and only if, the established care needs can be met at home by relatives, friends, and the community health agencies and services. This is true whether or not the patient is competent to state a preference for being at home. The responsibility for discharging the patient from an NHS facility now lies with the professional team, notably with the social worker appointed to carry out the community care assessment.

It is interesting to note that whilst other treatment decisions in palliative care can be made in partnership, the advent of the 'Community Care Act' in the United Kingdom has meant that the responsibility for discharge seems to lie entirely with the caring team. It is not truly a decision shared with the patient whose participation is limited to stating a preference for place of care, or taking full responsibility for self-discharge.

Thus patients who are at home cannot be removed against their (competent) choice but those in hospital cannot be discharged unless the professional team considers that they can be adequately cared for at home. It seems that 'position is nine-tenths of the law' in this respect, and it is this asymmetry in the patient's power to determine place of care which causes moral problems. Once in it, the patient's home is his castle—the problem lies in getting back home once in hospital!

For example, if a terminally ill man is at home and his wife states that she is no longer willing and/or able to provide the care which he needs and which cannot be provided entirely by the community services, then he cannot be removed from his home against his will unless he is shown to be incompetent. This is true even if professionals consider that he is not receiving the care he needs. In contrast, if he is in hospital and his wife indicates that she is unwilling and/or unable to provide that same level of care, then he cannot legally be discharged by the palliative care team. Although it could be said that he must have a right to be in his own home, he is effectively prevented from being discharged to it if it his spouse is unable or unwilling to undertake some aspects of care which are considered essential. In other words, when he is at home his wife (whose home it also is) has no say in whether he remains there, but when he is in hospital she can almost dictate whether he goes back to their shared home.

In fact it may happen that even if the care he needs at home can be provided by the community services, he may still not be discharged if she refuses to allow him home. This occurs because of the familiar internal conflict in the philosophy of palliative care which states that the unit of care is the 'whole family'. If one interprets this as meaning that his wife's interests are as important as the patient's, and if it does not seem in her interests for him to be at home (because of some associated physical effort and/or the inevitable emotional trauma), then the professional carers may well prevent him from going home by refusing to discharge him. Is this morally acceptable?

On balance it does seem harsh that the patient does not have a real part to play in deciding whether he can go home because this responsibility has been transferred to the carers by the Community Care Act. Ironically, this Act was passed in order to protect patients from precipitate and inappropriate discharge from hospital when their needs could not be met at home, but it has inevitably decreased patients' rights in terms of the normal discharge procedure.

It also seems unjustifiable that the needs of the patient's spouse should prevent him from being discharged. Yet this happens. Is there a morally preferable solution? This subject is discussed in Chapter 3.

We would suggest that it seems preferable to allow and encourage decisions about place of care to be made in the context of the decision-making partnership between the competent patient and carers. The availability of resources for care at home would obviously need to be considered, and this includes a frank discussion about the willingness and ability of relatives to undertake the often considerable demands of care. Ultimately it seems that the patient should be able to make the choice to go home, even if it is mutually acknowledged that the care the professionals consider essential may not be available there. If a competent patient can refuse life-prolonging and life-sustaining treatment or that which is required for symptom control, surely that same patient should be permitted to go home without taking the drastic measure of self-discharge, even if what others consider to be optimum care is not available at home.

9.4 Quality of care

Come, give us a taste of your
Shakespeare, *ı*

The basic ethos of palliative care has alwɑ
quality care for each individual patient.
difficult questions including: what does quality
measured, and who should measure it? The follow   ⌐of
quality encapsulates some important components   ⌐nie and
Calman 1994).

Quality is a concept which describes in both quantitative and qualitative
terms the level of care or services provided. Quality as a concept therefore
has two components. The first is quantitative and measurable, the second
is qualitative, though assessable, and associated with value judgements.
Quality is a relative not an absolute concept.

Quality is not therefore an analysis of activity. In describing the
quality of the palliative care service it must always be compared
to something else—either a similar activity or the same activity
measured at another time. It also implies measurable consistency
over time. Thus quality, as a relative concept, can always be
improved. This idea of continuous improvement is at the heart of all
quality initiatives.

Quality must be related to achievement of specific aims,
objectives, standards, and targets. Aims and objectives of palliative
care will require review but are unlikely to change radically, whereas
standards of care and targets will alter as knowledge and skills
increase and service provision alters to meet changing needs and as
available resources change.

Quality of palliative care is a multidimensional issue. It can be
seen to derive from six factors: professional knowledge, technical
skill, and competence; professional standards; attitudes and
behaviour (to patients); managerial functions; team work; teaching,
audit, and research.

There is considerable overlap between these headings, but for each
it is necessary to determine how quality should be assessed and who
should assess it. Professionals, patients, relatives, managers, and
other professionals may all be involved in objective and subjective
assessments of quality.

are two crucial principles governing quality initiatives in
ive care:

1. strive to do things right the first time
2. work for continual improvement.

We have said that quality must relate to the aims and objectives
of care. Quality is not just a matter of outcome, but is important at
all stages of delivery of palliative care. Those stages comprise input,
process, output, and outcome. Thus inputs of technology and human
resources must be of high calibre, which includes technical efficacy
and reliability, and professional knowledge and skills. The process of
care is in itself very beneficial to patients, but the quality of this
process is largely dependent on professional attitudes and behaviour
and team work. The quality of outputs in terms of symptom control, rehabilitation, emotional support, and so on is dependent on
professional knowledge and skills, but also on teaching, audit, and
research. High quality managerial functions are essential in providing the resources and environment which enable professionals to
provide high quality care.

In many areas of health care great emphasis is placed on the
assessment of quality in relation to outcomes. This requires an
ability to measure baseline and end-point states, whether in relation
to health, reassurance, satisfaction, or other effects. In palliative care
the baseline is in effect constantly moving as the illness changes the
patient's condition continuously. The final end-point at the conclusion of care is death, when existence on this earth ceases to have
any quality! Thus assessment of quality of outcome is very complex
in palliative care, because the outcome is quality of life and quality of
death for the patient, and the effect of the experience on the family.
Ideally, quality of life and of death can and should be assessed both
objectively and subjectively.

The person most able to assess overall quality of outcome is of
course the patient, but at the conclusion of the palliative care episode
the patient has usually died, so is not available to comment. It is
of very dubious benefit to rely on objective assessments by professionals and relatives only. Quality of life can be assessed by the
patient before the end of the episode, but it is difficult to separate the
influence of care from that of illness. For example, a falling quality
of life as measured on a scale may be more related to advancing
illness and dependency than to any aspect of care. Quality of life

assessments by patients are also very variable because they are by definition purely subjective. For example, some patients who can walk only 50 metres would regard their quality of life as very poor, whereas others who do not ascribe great importance to this factor might say that it was very good. The concept of quality of life and its inherent problems are further discussed in Chapter 14.

We would suggest that these considerable difficulties make quality of outcome difficult to assess sufficiently accurately and comprehensively to be useful, and that there is a moral obligation to spend at least as much time and effort evaluating quality of process and output, which can be more easily and reliably assessed and which are at least as relevant to overall quality of care as outcome.

We have earlier stressed that assessment of quality is both qualitative and quantitative. The latter can easily predominate to the almost total exclusion of the former, and this is not morally acceptable. It tends to happen because the principle of maximizing benefit (or utility) from palliative care resources commits us to setting targets, to auditing everything that can be audited, and many activities which cannot. Evaluation programmes, seen in this way under the umbrella of 'utility', require the introduction of measurement, and if there is going to be measurement there must be units of measurement. The consequence of this is that what is not in measurable units tends to be regarded as unimportant. Most of the benefits of palliative care do not come in measurable units, and so are not easily quantifiable, and thus the most important aspects of quality are all too readily marginalized. As a result of the desire to quantify (which is an implication of utility), there can be injustice in the evaluation of palliative care services.

Ethical aspects of the quality-determining factors of palliative care require further consideration.

9.4.1 *Knowledge, skills, and professional standards*

There is clearly an obligation on all health care professionals to improve knowledge and skills in the area of palliative care. It is much more contentious to say that managers too have ethical obligations here. No doubt some skills can be improved on the job, but many require time-out to be acquired, and staff must therefore be allowed study leave to attend courses and so on. Managers may reply that staff simply cannot be spared, but it may be argued that the requirement for study leave should be built into staffing levels. In so far as quality improvement derives from knowledge, then it will be slow to come unless staff can constantly upgrade their knowledge and skills.

The criteria for assessment of knowledge, skills, and competence are derived from other professionals. Appraisal is obviously an important quality initiative which should encourage any deficits to be rectified. A current difficulty in palliative care is the absence of appraisal for senior doctors. This could be a constructive process for both professional and personal development, thus contributing to quality of care.

9.4.2   *Attitudes and behaviour to patients*

We have stressed the fundamental importance of the attitude of beneficence, or a constant striving to assist the patient towards his or her total good, which is the aim of palliative care. The pursuance of the patient's total good necessarily entails respect for autonomy. In practice this means respecting the patients' informed choices as self-determining and self-governing beings. Attitudes of respect for autonomy and beneficence can be assessed by patients and professionals, but it is not plausible to suggest that a numerical value could be assigned to them. They can be assessed qualitatively but not quantitatively.

There are two interpretations of the idea of respect for autonomy, as we have already discussed (pp. 6–10) and the difference between them has radical implications for the ethics of palliative care and for the parameters by which quality of that care is judged. We have identified them as 'preference' autonomy and 'consumer' autonomy.

Autonomous choices or informed consent take place in the context of the professional consultation, where the patient retains the right of veto to unwanted treatment and the professional retains the right of veto to treatment professionally considered useless or harmful. The patient's informed choice as a self-determining and self-governing being is respected, as is the professional's choice of suitable treatments based on professional knowledge and skills. This interpretation of the idea of autonomy may be described as *preference* autonomy, and it is an integrated part of palliative care practice.

In recent years a different interpretation, that of *consumer* autonomy, has been proposed for application in the health care situation.
The idea of consumer autonomy underlies the free market economy
model of health care which has been recently introduced in the
United Kingdom. In the consumer interpretation of autonomy the
patient–professional role relationship is considered analogous to that
of a customer purchasing a product from a salesperson. The salesperson has no duty to refuse to sell goods considered inappropriate
to the customer if the latter insists on buying them.

As we have already indicated, if consumer ethics penetrate the
field of palliative care and replace traditional ethics, there will be
a fundamental change in the quality of palliative care in that its
very nature will be different. Moreover, different parameters, such
as whether patients and relatives wishes were granted in terms of
treatment, would be used for assessment of quality of care. We
suggest that if this happens the patients' total good will be less well
served than it currently is by the traditional ethics of palliative care.

9.4.3 Managerial functions and quality

There are two main sorts of managerial function and both raise
ethical issues: the management of resources and the management
of staff (or 'personnel' as managers no doubt call them). We consider the moral issues of resource allocation in a separate chapter.
Resource allocation, especially in terms of providing adequate
staffing levels in a structure which maximizes the benefits each staff
member can bring to the task, is a major quality issue. Procedures for
organizational audit have been developed as a way of assessing
quality in this area, and should be used in conjunction with objective
and subjective assessments by managers, clinical staff, patients, and
relatives.

The management of staff occurs in the context of the palliative
care team. It is fundamental to the concept of quality that the team is
able to measure its performance, and clinical audit provides a
medium to do this coupled with the procedure to improve quality of
care. Palliative care services which are multidisciplinary naturally
lend themselves to clinical audit on a team basis, rather than separate
medical and nursing audit. Since audit is now mandatory, this
quality initiative has become a fundamental part of clinical work in
palliative care. Once again there is a tendency to audit only those

factors which can be easily measured, whereas it is morally obligatory to audit also those factors essential to good care which can be assessed qualitatively but not quantitatively. Lack of a numerical evaluation should not exclude these factors from the audit process.

The team structure should enable staff to work together effectively and without unnecessary stress. It should also enable the clinical staff to have an input into both purchasing of health care and its provision. There should be adequate opportunity for discussion in management, so that staff feel able to support management decisions. If this is done, 'whistle-blowing' ought not to be undertaken without careful consideration.

The moral requirements of quality in teams indicate that there should be some way of dealing with conflict in the team. Providing such ways is an important function of management.

9.4.4   Research and audit

Research, development, and audit are central to and essential for the improvement of clinical practice in palliative care. New developments in treatment often raise new moral problems. Full evaluation of a new treatment, care policy, or procedure is morally required before it is adopted as standard practice so as to prevent ineffective, expensive, and possibly harmful treatment being used. Clinical audit and research serve different functions. Audit is the systematic analysis of the quality of clinical care and is based on existing standards and guidelines. Research looks at new procedures and takes care beyond that currently available. The practical and moral difficulties of conducting high quality research are discussed in the relevant chapter. There is a moral requirement to monitor the quality of research conducted.

The assessment of quality in palliative care is difficult and daunting, and this coupled with the knowledge that it is morally obligatory causes most clinical staff to approach it with some dread. This additional stress could be avoided, and important factors in care could be included in analysis to a greater extent than is currently the case, if quality assessments not based on numerical scales but based on a verbal scales such as bad, good, very good, and so on were more widely accepted. It is better to assess quality on a qualitative but not quantitative basis than not to assess it at all.

9.5 Conclusions

1. Patients' choices are respected, even if they are not fully autonomous nor perfectly competent, in order to preserve the principle of respect for autonomy in palliative care. Refusals of treatment are overruled only if there is no doubt that the patient is incompetent to make the decision.

2. Decisions regarding place of care should be made in the context of the partnership between patient and professional; caring relatives must be included in the discussion. Whilst relatives' interests must be considered by the patient, those interests should not undermine the patient's right to be at home.

3. There is a moral obligation to strive to improve quality of care. Some essential aspects of palliative care are not quantifiable in numerical terms; they must be assessed in qualitative terms which entails value judgements. It is not morally acceptable to omit them because they cannot be evaluated numerically.

10

Emotional care

*For some time, though, he struggled for more to hold on to.
'Are you sure you have told me everything you know about
his death?' he asked. I said, 'Everything'. 'It's not much, is
it?' I replied, 'but you can love completely without complete
understanding.' 'That I have known and preached,' my
father said.*

Norman Maclean, *A River Runs Through It*,
p. 159 (1976)

Health care workers involved with terminally ill patients have a
natural desire to alleviate their distress be it physical, psychological,
social, or spiritual. The entire ethos of palliative care is built on a
basic commitment to the relief of *all* distress or 'suffering'. A professional knowledge base and accompanying skills have developed
to deal with physical aspects of terminal illnesses and as a result
physical distress can be minimized or alleviated. A major component
of distress and suffering occurs in the mind, and derives from our
complex human nature as both individuals and social beings. We
have many interrelated emotional, social, and spiritual needs, which
if not met may give rise to distress and the experience of suffering.
Those working in palliative care are strongly motivated to reduce
this suffering, but at the same time realize that our ability to do so is
limited because we personally cannot meet the patients' emotional,
social, and spiritual needs. Therefore, we cannot bear the entire
responsibility for the patient's well-being in these areas. It is for this
reason that we have described the relief of emotional, psychological,
and social distress as extrinsic aims in palliative care. There are
many factors, both within and outside the patient, which are barriers
to wholeness, but however much we may want to influence all these
other factors we must accept that there are necessary practical and
philosophical limits to the scope of professional activity in palliative
care.

This does not mean that we will not do all in our power to alleviate this complex suffering, but rather that we acknowledge the limits of professional knowledge and skills, and explore the possibilities of relieving distress by means of ordinary human contact informed by our knowledge. In other words, we use our common humanity to comfort the patient, through the experience of companionship and that love we may call *agape*, in combination with giving advice based on the necessary and appropriate professional knowledge.

This is a controversial stance, for many will say that there is a separate and distinct set of professional skills and knowledge (called 'communication and counselling skills') which can be used to alleviate this suffering, but we would suggest that the application of the skills suggested does entail moral problems, and that perhaps we should focus instead on the gift of humanity which we share with our patients and strive to use that gift to alleviate some part of their suffering.

Discussion of psychosocial and spiritual care is difficult because it is an area in which many concepts merge and we are forced to confront and acknowledge both the complexity of our human nature and the limits of our ability to understand it. Our concepts of people as individuals and also as social beings merge—we see that personal well-being and relationships with others are inextricably mixed so that we cannot entirely separate the patient's welfare from that of relatives and friends. Therefore, we have a duty to alleviate the distress of relatives for the sake of the patient, and it may be argued that we also have a duty to alleviate the distress of relatives for their own sake (see Chapter 3, p. 70). Psychological, social, and spiritual distress are seen to be inextricably mixed. The roles of professional carers all merge and overlap as all are concerned with the patient's suffering. Normal psychological responses to terminal illness merge with responses we regard as abnormal and indicative of mental illness requiring psychotropic drugs and the expertise of a psychiatrist. The expression of distress merges with the relief of that distress, as when giving expression to anger helps to alleviate it, and so assessment of needs merges with interventions to meet those needs. Finally, ideas of ordinary professional competence merge with ideas of communication skills and suggested specific counselling skills, giving rise to confusion!

Despite the fact that so many of the margins we use in separating concepts for the purposes of discussion become very blurred in this area, it is still possible and necessary to explore the moral issues which arise in our attempts to alleviate psychological, social, and spiritual pain. Pain of this nature may be described broadly for our present purposes as 'suffering'. Care directed at the relief of this suffering is often seen as inevitably or necessarily morally good, just as pain control may be regarded as morally good. However, it is apparent that the ways in which pain control is carried out may be morally good or bad, justifiable or unjustifiable, and so the morality of the process of pain control must be examined. It is not sufficient to say that pain control is intrinsically good, so that all ways of carrying it out must be good and right! In the same way, we can say that whilst attempting to alleviate psychological, social, and spiritual distress may be morally good, the morality of the process of relieving that distress must be examined. Whilst the motivation to relieve this suffering is good, the process of care used may be morally good or bad, justifiable or unjustifiable.

Since there has been a tendency to regard all psychological, social, and spiritual care as morally good, such care has not been exposed to the moral scrutiny which we apply to medical interventions such as investigation and treatment. This situation is morally unsatisfactory because it leads to unconditional approbation of all attempts to relieve mental aspects of suffering and to the uncritical use of methods which may be morally wrong, either because they entail unjustifiable infringements of autonomy, or because their harms outweigh their benefits, or because they consume an unjustifiable portion of resources. Instead we should examine the morality of our approach to these aspects of care, and this can be done be using a format roughly parallel to that used for care relating to the physical aspects of the illness. This is appropriate because the same moral principles apply to psychological, social, and spiritual care as to physical care. Moral judgement is not suspended simply because our care is directed at non-physical aspects of the patient's well-being or because our goal is the removal of psychosocial barriers to wholeness!

We therefore discuss issues of consent to care, communication, and assessment of psychosocial and spiritual status and needs, and decisions regarding interventions. This provides a comprehensive framework which is familiar and easily understood by those providing other aspects of palliative care. It should be stressed that this discussion relates to the morality of the process of care, and is not intended to be a description of the care itself.

10.1 Consent to psychosocial and spiritual care

Palliative care workers meet the patient in the context of a terminal illness. It is this illness which caused the patient to seek help, and so it is this illness for which the patient has given implied consent for health care. The scope of such implied consent is difficult to define, but it suffices to say that we cannot assume that a patient implicitly consents to whatever care interventions the professionals consider are appropriate. Someone asking for pain control does not necessarily want to explore feelings related to the diagnosis, let alone those related to previous life crises, close relationships, or sexuality! It is disrespectful of patient autonomy to embark on personal discussions unless the patient has indicated a desire or at least willingness to do so.

Of course patients may want help with social, psychological, or spiritual problems, especially once physical distress has been alleviated and life is no longer dominated by discomfort. It is obviously appropriate to ask frequently what problems the patient wants to address, and if an area of distress is apparent to carers they may ask the patient if their perceptions are accurate and if discussion of the problem is wanted. It is not morally acceptable to assume that the patient wants and consents to care for emotional, social, and spiritual distress, and therefore to instigate deeply personal assessments and interventions.

This is a difficult moral issue in palliative care, where carers are so strongly motivated towards the relief of all distress that they may tend to assume that the patient, in consenting to give a history of the illness and in permitting physical care and examination, is also consenting to give a personal life history and is permitting detailed assessment of psychosocial status and problems. This is surely not the case, and therefore the assumption of consent is not morally justifiable. Since the patient is very vulnerable in the patient–carer relationship, such assumptions may lead to the infliction of 'care' on the patient who may find it difficult to refuse this care or even to escape from it, especially if it is 'sold' to the patient in a package in which it is inextricably mixed with physical care and treatment which *is* wanted.

For example, if a patient knows that the person providing access to much needed and wanted symptom control also probes deeply into emotional matters, the patient will feel obliged to tolerate such probing in order to obtain the benefits of symptom control. Most would consider that it is not morally justifiable to bind different aspects of care together in this way so that it is difficult for the patient to select those which they want and to refuse those which they do not want. Yet this is so often done by health care workers in the context of palliative care that they cease to be aware that they are binding the two aspects of care together.

Even if carers appreciate that the patient has not consented to a personal discussion, deeply personal questioning is sometimes said to be justifiable because psychosocial and spiritual care are seen as good in themselves, as being inextricably linked to physical welfare, and as being part of the remit of the palliative care team—in other words as 'intrinsic' to palliative care. Indeed, all members of the team may come to think that they have failed in their professional duty if they have not explored the patient's feelings and made attempts to alleviate mental distress.

We would argue that psychosocial care is extrinsic to palliative care and that it should be offered to patients but not inflicted or forced upon them by well-meaning professionals. It is definitely a matter for consent. The question 'how did you feel about so and so ...' is not necessarily morally acceptable, since it is intrusive if the patient does not in fact want to talk about feelings but may find it difficult to refuse in the context of the interview. Instead it is morally preferable to ask 'would you like to talk about how you felt about so and so ...' , and to offer to discuss any areas of distress the patient may perceive.

There is a subtle but morally important distinction between encouraging patients to talk about their feelings and asking searching question which it is difficult to avoid answering. We suggest that more consideration should be given to the moral justification for asking questions to which it is difficult to reply without divulging deeply personal information. Whilst many patients want to talk about their feelings, not all do and they should not be placed in situations from which it is difficult to escape without making personal revelations.

10.2   Communication of thoughts and emotions

Communication skills are said to be important in assessing the patient's emotional state and in elucidating needs. Communication is of course a two-way process—it is about receiving as well as giving; moral issues arising from the giving of information to patients have been discussed, but in this chapter the process of gaining information from the patient is particularly relevant. It gives rise to moral issues which have received less attention in palliative care.

Communication is the major vehicle of human understanding, and consequently it is of enormous moral and practical importance and so has been much studied. These studies have revealed a set of behaviours which are said to facilitate good communication, and this set of behaviours is often taught as 'communication skills'.

The application of any artificially produced behaviours to the area of communication is morally problematic; our relationships to each other are so important—in so many ways they are 'all we have got', and these relationships are so dependent on honest and open communication that any attempt to manipulate communication or to dissemble in the process must be exposed to moral scrutiny. Any intent to deceive in communication stands in need of moral justification, whatever the relationship of the parties involved.

The relationship of people to each other is important in determining the nature of communication which is most appropriate. The subtleties of disclosure of thoughts and emotions between people in different relationships to each other are highly relevant and more than a little problematic in palliative care. It is important to appreciate the practical and philosophical differences between personal and professional relationships, whilst at the same time acknowledging that in palliative care patients and professionals sometimes pass between the two. This transfer from the professional to the personal relationship can be of benefit to both patient and professional, but it carries emotional risks to both, and a high potential emotional cost to the carer. Much may be achieved, but with less risk, by remaining within the context of a professional relationship, and this is in fact what happens in the majority of patient–carer contacts.

Deeply personal relationships which occur between spouses, sexual partners, close friends, and within families entail great openness but also great vulnerability. The strength of the bonds of affection and trust in the strength of those bonds enable friends to communicate ideas about the world and, more importantly, about each other. Thoughts and emotions are communicated freely and honestly. Long-term attachment combined with this free exchange of personal thoughts often enables substantial mutual understanding which develops slowly over time. Ultimately, in the closest of relationships each party becomes sensitive to the emotions of the other and has some true understanding of what the other is experiencing and perhaps even of the meaning of that experience for the other. Positive and loving thoughts and emotions are communicated freely and shared.

Deep attachment at a personal level also permits the sharing of pain and mutual disapproval. A close relationship is not one of unconditional positive regard—we are and ought to be critical of each other, and if we are to be genuine in our responses to each other then it must be possible to express disapproval as well as approbation. This is possible precisely because of the security of the underlying bond of affection which is mutually understood and acknowledged, and because it is possible and morally desirable to continue to love someone whilst disapproving of some of their attitudes and actions—'loving the sinner whilst hating the sin'. Thus only people who are deeply attached at a personal level can withstand the impact of the communication of full awareness of disapproval from the other. Often even in the closest of relationships the full extent of disapproval and perhaps associated anger is not communicated for the good moral reason that its impact could be personally destructive to the other, or out of a natural gentleness towards the other. Many people appreciate that we are most vulnerable towards those we most love. Nonetheless, judgements about behaviour are expressed in the confidence that mutual loyalty and trust in the affection which underpins the relationship will enable the judgement to be heard without threatening the bond.

In contrast, those less deeply attached but wanting to maintain and develop friendship will not usually communicate the full extent of negative feelings towards the other, in order not to threaten the relationship and because of uncertainty about the effect of disapproval on the other. In contrast, positive feelings are usually communicated freely.

The relationship of the professional to a patient in the context of palliative care is different from a personal friendship. In the patient–carer relationship an attitude of beneficence on behalf of the professional, trust in that beneficence on behalf of the patient, and mutual respect for autonomy all constitute the bond and determine its nature. Thus the professional communicates information which the patient wants with sensitivity and gentleness, so as not to harm the patient with truth communicated brutally. The professional has a duty to give advice with regard to treatment, based on knowledge of the disease, previous patients, and this particular patient, and also has a duty to advise the patient of lifestyles harmful to personal health or to the health of others (for example, risks for sexual contacts of HIV positive patients).

It is generally considered that the professional will not be morally judgemental of the patient, but it must be said that where the patient's behaviour is harming those around him, especially those responsible for care, then it seems appropriate for the professional to point this out. In this regard the patient is simply being treated as a responsible person with the ability to govern his own behaviour. Disapproval of the patient as a person is not expressed, nor is gratuitous disapproval of attitudes or behaviour not immediately relevant to health, because to do so would be to jeopardize the relationship and thus possibly sabotage its purpose. The relationship is not a deeply personal one which could be expected to withstand the expression of such disapproval. Indeed it would probably be construed as personal rejection by the patient whose trust in the professional might then be impaired. One might say that in the professional relationship the judgemental attitude is appropriately inhibited, whilst acknowledging that this inevitably entails a cost in terms of some loss of the genuine, human, and personal aspects of the interaction.

Since an attitude of beneficence arising from a strong motivation to act in accordance with the patient's total good is fundamental to the professional role, it is natural for those involved in palliative care to be concerned for the patient's emotional welfare. This professional concern will naturally manifest itself in appropriate verbal and non-verbal communication with the patient, who will then be aware of that concern. Any deficiency in the carer's attitude of concern is a deficiency of professional conduct, and it is likely to show itself in insensitive and/or ineffective communication with the patient.

If an attitude of concern is morally appropriate and required in palliative care, and if such an attitude is naturally communicated verbally and non-verbally, is there really a need for the teaching of 'communication skills'? If the carer's attitude is deficient or inappropriate, is it morally justifiable to conceal this beneath a mask of behaviour patterns or skills which the carer has been trained to use so that the patient thinks the carer is concerned? We would argue that concealment of a deficient attitude by the deliberate use of verbal and non-verbal techniques which normally demonstrate concern constitutes intent to deceive the patient, and is not morally justifiable. This is a contentious position to adopt, but some examples help to illustrate the moral problems and adverse consequences associated with the inappropriate use of a set behaviour patterns called 'communication skills'.

Carers may be taught to adopt a bodily posture of attention, with eyes at the same level as the patient's, and to maintain eye contact. Of course, a carer with the appropriate attitude of concern would naturally adopt a position in which a quiet discussion feels comfortable, and in listening to the patient would maintain a natural degree of eye contact. The practical disadvantage of teaching carers techniques of position like this is that they become aware of non-verbal behaviour which is normally unconscious, spontaneous, and honest. They may then develop a stilted style which appears unnatural and unconvincing, and they may become incapable of spontaneous and honest non-verbal interaction. The moral disadvantage is that the patient may be deceived by false and artificial non-verbal signals into believing that a carer who is not actually listening or concerned is attending to every word. Fortunately, patients are very perceptive and soon realize the behaviour is not genuine.

Carers may also be taught to demonstrate frequently to the patient that they are really listening and that what is said is appreciated. It is suggested that repeating two or three words from the patient's last sentence may achieve this, or that paraphrasing the sentence will demonstrate that it was understood. The practical risk is that the carer will sound like an echo, or that the patient will be puzzled and perhaps frustrated by repetition of statements. The moral problem is that once again the intention may be to demonstrate concern manifested in dedicated listening when in fact the carer is not feeling concerned at all, or to demonstrate understanding when in fact the carer cannot understand the patient's experience and emotions, or their meaning for the patient.

What is important is that the carer does have an appropriate attitude, not that the patient thinks the carer has this attitude. If the carer's attitude is deficient or inappropriate, the whole patient–carer interaction will not yield a morally acceptable outcome because the behaviour of the carer in the decision-making partnership and in treatment is likely to be defective. Deceiving the patient into thinking that the carer's attitude is one of beneficence combined with respect cannot ensure the desired outcome of the relationship. We therefore conclude that it is the correct moral basis of the relationship which should be taught and emphasized to carers, and only the small minority who have atypical or unusual verbal or non-verbal communication patterns should be taught communication skills in order that their responses may be better understood by patients.

Communication in psychosocial care and spiritual care is directed towards the expression of the patients' thoughts and emotions, and patients should feel appropriately assured that the carers have a proper professional concern for their welfare, and so are genuinely listening and trying to understand.

It is inevitable that as carers and patients come to know each other, personal friendship may develop in a minority of contacts, with the expected subtle but important alterations in the nature of communication. Whilst there are many mutual gains to be made from this change, the emotional costs to the carer in terms of shared emotional trauma and eventual loss are high, and relationships of personal friendship with the majority of patients would not be sustainable by carers. It is not morally justifiable to subject carers to continuous emotional trauma by expecting them to conduct their relationships with patients at the level of personal friendship because the damage done to the carers would be unacceptably great. Such damage is not justified by any (possible) benefit to patients. Rather, the expectation should be of appropriate professional concern, which only exceptionally may stray beyond those bounds into the realms of personal friendship.

10.3   Assessment of psychosocial and spiritual status

Since the context of palliative care is that of terminal illness and ultimate death, emotional reactions to the changes of illness and future losses are expected and have a major impact on patient welfare, with which the professional is concerned. It is therefore appropriate for carers to want some information about psychosocial factors. The moral problem is that in current palliative care philosophy it is recommended that a great deal of information is required to make an adequate assessment, and one wonders how this can be obtained without subjecting all but the most open and talkative patients to an intrusive barrage of questions.

For example, the Oxford Textbook of Palliative Medicine (Doyle *et al*, 1994, p. 566) describes psychosocial assessment of the *individual* as follows:

In assessing the individual we need to establish what changes the illness has wrought, as well as who they are. We need to know how their life has changed since the illness and who or what currently supports them. We need to understand their reaction to the illness and its implications for them. We need to identify any practical or emotional unfinished business they may have. Assessing practical issues will lead us on to values and beliefs. Does the individual see their illness as a punishment? How have they dealt with crises in the past?

In addition, information might be sought about deeply personal matters such as the patient's spiritual concerns and sexuality.

Assessment of the family is also considered essential:

In order to assess the strengths and difficulties of a family and its members, we need to understand how it works. We must discover the normal patterns of communication, support and conflict in the family, and the extent to which they have been disrupted by illness ... The history of the current family and their individual experiences within their previous families will be significant factors in their ability to cope with the present crisis.

Further assessment of the family's physical resources and social network in the community is also regarded as essential.

It is obvious that a great deal of information is considered necessary for this assessment. On what moral grounds is it being sought? It is suggested that a detailed assessment such as this is the best way to plan *interventions* which will ultimately benefit the patient. Detailed questioning which is likely to be intrusive may constitute a harm, and if it is to be morally justified there must be a reasonable likelihood of moderate benefit derived from psychosocial intervention. The benefit derived from such interventions is difficult to evaluate and probably impossible to distinguish from the benefit which patients appear to gain from talking about their situation and problems to a concerned but non-judgemental professional. Presumably this latter benefit, which is related to the ability to talk freely to another, could also be gained without the possible harms of intrusive questioning by the simple willingness of the professional to listen in a sympathetic and non-judgemental manner. Such listening would be entirely appropriate to the professional–patient relationship in the context of palliative care. It therefore seems difficult to justify intrusive and potentially exhausting questioning on the grounds that it is necessary to plan interventions which are in themselves difficult to evaluate. In contrast, those patients and families who show willingness to participate in a full assessment which is carried out respectfully will not be harmed and benefit is likely.

Professionals should not put pressure on families to divulge personal information (which they would rather withhold) on the grounds that it is 'for the patient's good'. Families are entitled to keep confidences, and may not want to talk about and relive past crises and describe how they were resolved. For example, a family who have previously lost a child may not want to talk about the experience and how they coped with it. They might find such a conversation an unwelcome intrusion which reawakened distressing memories at a time when they did not wish to have to confront them and relive them by describing them to a health care professional involved in care related to a new illness.

What is important is that patients must be able to choose the extent to which they participate in psychosocial assessments just as they choose which investigations they wish to undergo and the extent to which they participate in decision making. Pressure should not be put on either patient or family to reveal that which they would prefer to keep private. Moreover, those who do not wish to divulge personal information should not be labelled as 'withdrawn' or 'isolated' or described rather patronizingly as 'in need of their own defences'. Even in palliative care there must be some right to privacy!

10.4   Assessment of psychosocial needs

We all have emotional, psychological, social, and spiritual needs which if not met can give rise to suffering. These needs are usually met by the patient's lifestyle and contact with friends and relatives. They are not normally met by contact with health care workers. Contact with those involved in palliative care is important to many patients and can go some way to relieving loneliness, isolation, and a sense of worthlessness. It may also partially meet a need for concern and physical contact from others. Nevertheless, contact with carers, whilst being helpful, is not normally sufficient, and it cannot replace interaction with friends and relatives. In other words, professional carers cannot personally meet all the emotional, psychological, social, and spiritual needs of the patient and it is unreasonable to expect them to try.

It must be stressed that unmet emotional, psychological, and spiritual needs can be identified only by the patient, and not by carers. There is a danger that carers assume some unmet needs on the basis of their own experience, values, and beliefs. They may then consider it necessary to explore in detail those perceived or assumed needs which the patient may hitherto be unaware of (and therefore not distressed by) or which the patient may not wish to discuss. For example, a carer may suggest to a patient that she has an unmet need for continuing sexual contact. The patient, whose libido is reduced by hormone therapy and illness, may not perceive this need but may be very suggestible and may also consider that as a normal woman she 'ought' to have this need. In fact it may be very difficult for her to have sexual contact for many reasons. Thus an iatrogenic unmet need may be generated and associated distress may result. Harm may also be caused to the patient by intrusive questioning.

The patient may also be harmed if the carer concludes, rightly or wrongly, that the patient's response to circumstances derives from some deep-seated 'hang-up' or unfinished emotional business which the carer considers the patient 'needs' to sort out. In fact the patient may be too exhausted or simply unwilling to confront a long-term 'hang-up' which was not faced and dealt with even in health. There is a definite risk that the patient may be distressed by being encouraged or persuaded to confront a traumatic issue, and there is a further serious risk that the patient's condition may deteriorate whilst this issue is unresolved and the patient is in a transitional state of even greater distress, confusion, or anxiety. This may result in unnecessary trauma which the patient is unable to deal with, and an excessively traumatic death amidst relived distress may result. Carers are morally bound to make every attempt to prevent such an unfortunate outcome.

Denial of the diagnosis or prognosis by the patient may be perceived by carers as a need to break down that denial. Since denial is a protective mechanism, there is a significant risk that the patient may be harmed if it is broken down. This risk is therefore justifiable only if the denial is causing the patient to refuse essential treatment or if it is in itself causing emotional distress. It is not morally justifiable to risk harm to the patient by breaking down denial for the sake of the relatives or carers.

A more difficult philosophical question is whether sadness, anxiety, and a sense of loss in a terminal illness constitute or represent any sort of unmet need, or whether they are simply appropriate human responses. If the latter is the case, then it is doubtful if the patient would benefit from their abolition, even if that was wanted and was possible. It seems to make little sense to say that such sadness, loss, and appropriate worry are in any way 'needs' which should be met, or to say that they are inappropriate responses which should be reduced or manipulated in some way into alternative responses which carers consider more beneficial.

On the other hand, fear, some forms of anxiety, and guilt because of an underlying assumption that the illness is in some way the patient's fault may represent a need for more information which the professional is able to give, and by so doing can offer genuine (but not false) reassurance.

In general, the purposes of assessing unmet needs must be to benefit the patient simply by listening and acknowledging their importance, and where possible to stimulate others to meet those needs. It is obviously morally problematic to try to make friends and family relate to the patient in a certain way so as to meet the needs identified, since those friends and family must consent to manipulation of their behaviour in this way. Indeed they might find such suggestions impertinent, patronizing, or intrusive, and their perception of the patient's emotional needs may be different from that of the professional carers. Whilst a sensitive and tactful approach may be effective, the risks of harm to both family and patient are high.

As always in palliative care, a delicate balance has to be struck between the harms, risks, and benefits of all care options, even those intended to alleviate emotional suffering.

10.5   Interventions in psychosocial and spiritual care

It is necessary to consider exactly what the carers are doing in undertaking this form of care. Having determined the activities involved it is then important to decide whether they fall outside the sphere of professional expertise which one can reasonably expect of those involved in palliative care, and if other skills are required. If the latter is the case, then there is a strong moral obligation to acquire those skills.

Perhaps the most important activity, although it can scarcely be described as an intervention, is genuine listening with an attempt at understanding, motivated by professional concern for the patient's welfare. We have earlier said that if the carer's attitude is correct, then appropriate verbal and non-verbal behaviour in the role of listener will follow, and training to follow a pre-set pattern of behaviour called 'communication skills' will be at best unhelpful and at worst harmful.

Giving information is also an important intervention. Patients continue to need information throughout their illness, and this need is met from the carers' professional knowledge base. Information may be required about a wide range of topics such as financial assistance and domiciliary services, common symptoms, or modes of death, or how to tell the children about a terminal illness, and part of the professionals' skill lies in giving this information when needed and in a sensitive manner. Patients sometimes need reassurance that a certain emotion which they or those close to them are feeling is normal. Giving information is definitely part of the professional role, and one would expect carers to be competent in this area. The required knowledge base, experience, normal human sensitivity, and the appropriate attitude towards the patient will ensure that this need is met. Once again, no special expertise distinct from that which the health care professional should possess is required.

Psychiatric or psychotherapeutic interventions such as drug treatments for depression and anxiety, training in relaxation and visualization techniques, and cognitive–behavioural techniques may be required for those patients who are depressed rather than sad, overwhelmed by inappropriate anxiety, or suffering from psychoses or temporary confusional states. In the course of their work carers will be expected to recognize a patient's need for expert advice and intervention.

Sometimes patients and families seem to lack the confidence to make decisions and to act. It is suggested that their confidence can be increased enabling them to address their problems by simple measures such as reminding them of their resources and strengths, encouraging them to identify their problems, and using professional knowledge about the illness to help them set realistic goals. None of these activities would seem to require special training, nor do they represent some form of distinct professional expertise. Once again an attitude of respect for autonomy and a desire to help, combined with professional knowledge, sensitivity, and common sense, would seem to be sufficient.

Patients and families may have difficulty communicating amongst themselves in the emotionally charged circumstances of palliative care. Some carers, particularly social workers, undertake to overcome barriers to communication by being present at a family gathering and ensuring that every member of the family hears a complete story about the illness. Members may be encouraged to talk about their reaction to the information so that there is a shared awareness of feelings. It is suggested that the presence of a 'skilled outsider, the carer, can provide the security and control which family members feel they need to release their emotions' (Doyle *et al*, 1994).

It is obvious that setting up such an important and emotionally charged meeting requires judgement and sensitivity (as well as explanation to all family members and consent to the activity), and that the carer must be able to exercise some control over the proceedings to prevent family members harming each other by disclosures of dislike or disapproval which may be rooted deep in historical family conflict. It would seem that conducting such a delicate interview with such in-built potential for disaster probably does require special training. In order to prevent harm and gain benefit from family therapy of this nature, training is mandatory; those who feel sufficiently confident and ambitious to intervene in the affairs of patient and family in this way should not do so unless they have the appropriate experience in family therapy. This can be gained from the areas of psychiatry and psychotherapy where much has been learned about influencing family interaction.

In summary, we might say that relief of psychosocial and spiritual distress by carers is as much a matter of 'being' as of 'doing'; it is about the people that they are rather than about what they actually do. They need to be fully developed and understanding people who have a genuine professional concern for the patient coupled with the necessary professional knowledge. In general, no mystical or special expertise is required.

10.6 Counselling and counselling skills

The meaning of the term 'counselling' has become blurred by its many different uses. The British Association for Counselling states that the counselling task is to give the client a chance to explore, discover, and clarify ways of living more satisfyingly and resource-fully. It is said that clients attending counsellors want 'real people who are prepared to meet them emotionally, who will listen to them and hear what they say. They want people who have a genuine concern for them and now share with them their thoughts and ideas. They want a partnership in which power is shared.' (Rogers, 1969).

It is suggested that there are universally applicable or transferable skills which can be acquired from professional courses and which enable their possessors to have insights denied to the uninitiated into the human experience. It is further suggested that the application of these skills (but with deliberate avoidance of giving direction or advice) enables the client to solve personal problems. If such distinct professional knowledge and skills exist, then one must ask if it is morally appropriate to apply them in the palliative care area. If it is, then there is a moral obligation for carers to acquire them.

The idea that counselling is a professional activity seems paradoxical in the light of the client's aims and desires. The paradox is that if clients want 'real people' and 'genuine concern' for themselves individually and personally, they cannot want a professional service for which there is training. It makes no sense to speak of being *trained* to *be genuine*. It might be possible to train someone to appear genuine, but not to be genuine. The very concepts of a *client* and a *professional* are incompatible with a *personal* relationship which entails a genuine personal concern. We have stressed that a personal relationship is different from the profes-sional–client relationship. To have genuine personal concern is one thing, and a thing for which there (logically) can be no training, whereas to have professional skills is another thing, and a thing for which there can be training. Counselling of the non-directive kind tries to combine the two and therefore it has a contradiction built into it.

Three concepts lie at the heart of counselling theory, practice, and training, and all are problematic in that they may be unrealistic and even contrary to our experience of human relationships. These are empathy, congruence, and unconditional positive regard.

Empathy is usually described as the ability to understand and share the emotions of the other person so as to enter their private perceptual world, and to live in that world without making judgements. It entails understanding the meaning that emotions and experience have for the other. It is doubtful if even very close friends can achieve this level of understanding, which certainly cannot be acquired on a fee-paying sessional basis with fixed time constraints.

A non-judgemental approach is also incompatible with genuineness because we are and ought to be at least critical of each other— we need the comments and reactions of others to govern our own behaviour. We have acknowledged that in the professional–patient relationship some degree of genuine and personal response is sacrificed because it is necessary to inhibit the judgemental attitude. One cannot undertake to be both genuine and non-judgemental.

The concept of unconditional positive regard poses similar problems; we do not have positive regard for persons *regardless* of what they do. Whilst we refrain from voicing judgements in the professional relationship, that does not mean that we unconditionally approve of everything the patient does and says. In personal relationships the friend is held in high regard but this is influenced by behaviour, and judgements are expressed in more or less explicit ways. True unconditional positive regard does not exist in either personal or professional relationships and it seems to stretch credibility to ask us to believe that it can exist in an artificial 'counselling' relationship. Would such an artificial relationship be morally desirable anyway?

What can and should exist in personal and professional relationships is respect for the other as a self-determining and self-governing person, who has intrinsic worth as a human being. This does not equate with unconditional positive regard for all attitudes and conduct.

The idea of congruence poses similar moral problems; a person is said to be congruent when he is accurately aware of what he is experiencing, and when he communicates to another fully and honestly exactly what he is experiencing. There are several difficulties with this idea. Firstly, it is not always possible to be sure what one is thinking or experiencing in a given situation because our motives and emotions can be inaccessible. One need not be a Freudian to see this. Secondly, if congruence is 'being what you are' at all levels of feeling and awareness, and then communicating exactly that to the other, then there is surely a risk of bringing a relationship (whether personal or professional) to an abrupt, unsatisfactory, and possibly destructive end. People would need to be deeply attached at a personal level to withstand the full blast of congruence! Indeed, in the context of the carer–patient relationship it would not be acceptable to be congruent, since this might entail expressing strong disapproval, or considerable but inappropriate affection, or worse still sexual attraction! It is simply not morally acceptable to be congruent in the carer–patient relationship, and it would not seem logically possible to be simultaneously non-judgemental and congruent in the 'counselling' relationship.

In summary, we might say that it seems logically impossible to combine these proposed 'counselling skills' in any human relationship. It also seems morally unacceptable to attempt to introduce them into the carer–patient relationship of palliative care. Indeed, patients would probably be harmed by carers becoming enmeshed in role conflicts through attempting to be a counsellor (which is obviously a specific contract relationship) as well as a nurse, doctor, social worker, chaplain, and so on.

It is morally preferable to maintain appropriate attitudes in the carer–patient relationship rather than to adopt the artificial postures and set behaviour patterns which communication and counselling skills can so easily become.

10.7 Conclusions

1. Psychosocial and spiritual care must be subjected to moral scrutiny in the same way as physical care; consent must be sought and the potential harms and risks of care must be balanced against potential benefits.

2. Genuine professional concern for the patients' welfare will naturally lead to effective communication; the gift of ordinary human companionship informed by professional knowledge goes some way to alleviating psychosocial and spiritual distress and loneliness.

3. Artificially acquired sets of behaviour such as communication skills and counselling skills may inhibit spontaneous communication, are likely to cause role conflict, and may entail a degree of deceit on behalf of the carer. The specific contractual counselling role is inappropriate for professional–patient contact in palliative care.

4. Palliative care needs well-developed, wise, and compassionate people, whose common sense is combined with professional knowledge; it does not need people who lack these characteristics but are trained to appear as if they possess them.

11 ....

Research

Oh! let us never, never doubt
What nobody is sure about!
Hilaire Belloc, *The Microbe* from *Cautionary Tales* (1907)

Why does research in palliative medicine give rise to ethical problems? Let us begin by considering why research can give rise to ethical problems in any branch of medicine.

11.1 Codes of ethics

The problem is stated in the 'Declaration of Helsinki' which was adopted by the eighteenth World Medical Association in 1964 and revised by the World Medical Assembly in 1975, 1983, and 1989. The Declaration of Helsinki introduces the problem by quoting from the Declaration of Geneva the key phrase 'The health of my patient will be my first consideration'. Biomedical research will at some stage require experimentation involving human subjects and it can be pointed out that, in so far as this is research, it is by its nature concerned with objectives other than the health of the subject—namely, reaching conclusions about the effectiveness of some therapy. It could of course be replied at this point that the Declaration of Geneva does not say that the health of the patient should be the doctor's *only* consideration; just that it should be the primary consideration. In developing this reply we must remember that some research is what is often called 'therapeutic'. In other words, there may be situations in which a range of possible therapies have been tried on a given patient and not found to be very effective, and the doctor therefore wishes to try out a new and perhaps untested therapy. In such a situation it can be argued that the health of the patient remains the primary consideration but not the only consideration. The doctor may obtain results of a nature which may be helpful to future patients.

As we shall see when we come to the special problems of research in the palliative area, this reply may not satisfy everyone involved in palliative medicine. But before we move on to the special problems in the palliative field we must note that the reply does not fit the large area of non-therapeutic research. Non-therapeutic research by its nature is not directed towards the health of present patients but towards the establishment of scientific conclusions which may benefit future patients—but may also actually harm the patients on whom the research is presently being conducted. But of course medical science must have progress and new therapies must be tested against the existing ones. Hence, there is a conflict within the reasonable objectives of medicine—to give patients the best known treatments and to make continuous efforts to replace the best known treatments with better ones. This conflict could be stated as one between, on the one hand, the principles of beneficence and non-maleficence, of helping and not harming the patient, and on the one hand, of utility, of improving the general level of available therapies. Let us look in more detail at this dilemma

11.2   Randomized double-blind controlled trials

If we wish to demonstrate that some proposed new treatment is a cause of improvement (or indeed of harmful side-effects) the proposed treatment must be compared with the conventional treatment or with the giving of a placebo. The hope is that there will be a higher rate of improvement or care in the experimental group than in the control group, and that the results will be statistically significant, or large enough to rule out the possibility that the difference occurred as a result of chance variation. Moreover, it is not sufficient to rule out the 'chance' possibility; it must be possible to rule out that the result is due to other factors, such as the severity of the illness, or the age of the patients, or some other factor prior to the treatment. It is argued by proponents of randomized trials that by assigning a large number of subjects randomly to the experimental or the control group other possible factors will be ruled out. And since neither the patients nor the participating researchers know who has been given the new and who the conventional treatment or placebo there can be no psychological effects influencing the results. Some trials try to deal with the extraneous factors by matching the samples for age, severity of illness, and so on, but it is argued that it is difficult to be sure that all variables have been matched. Randomization, it is claimed, matches for all variables.

So far we have simply outlined a research method. Ethical issues enter the picture if it is further argued that this is the most effective method and that therefore there is a moral obligation to use it to ensure the safety of future patients.

There are, however, ethical problems attached to this methodology. As we have seen there are ethical obligations to help and not to harm patients. Let us combine these for present purposes and speak of the 'therapeutic obligation'. Now consider a randomized control trial (RCT), not double-blind, to establish the superiority or otherwise of two treatments, A and B. We can stipulate that at the beginning of the RCT there is no clear evidence of the superiority of either A or B. The methodology in that case would suggest that patients could be randomly assigned to each 'arm' of the study without violating the therapeutic obligation. If by the conclusion of the experiments it emerged that we could be 90 per cent certain that treatment A was superior to B, we would have a persuasive scientific outcome. The difficulty is, however, that we could have drawn the same conclusion at some earlier point when, say, we were 75 per cent certain of the outcome. Now trends can reverse themselves, so 75 per cent certainty would not be so acceptable scientifically; nevertheless the majority of clinicians faced with that figure would be persuaded to switch their patients to the new therapy. In other words, the ethical obligation to obtain a convincing scientific result may conflict with the therapeutic obligation to do the best possible for a given group of patients. Moreover, in the case given it was stipulated that the doctor does not have a view at the start of the trial which of the therapies is likely to be the more effective. But in most cases the doctor will have some notion which is the more effective. In such a case it is not clear that the RCT can get going at all without violating the therapeutic obligation. A major scientific method for advancing knowledge seems therefore to conflict with a major ethical obligation. This is the classic ethical dilemma, since there seem to be disadvantages in accepting either of the alternatives.

There have been many ingenious attempts at solving the dilemma, but they tend to fall into one or other of two sorts. The first group of arguments try to deny that the dilemma is real. It is said that if we properly understand the nature of the RCT and the therapeutic obligation, we shall see that the two are fully compatible. The second group accept the reality of the ethical dilemma and make suggestions as to how harm to the patients may be minimized. Let us look briefly at one attempt to deny the reality of the dilemma.

This attempt to deny the reality of the dilemma involves a procedural move. It might be argued that the dilemma arises only because we are expecting one and the same group of people to act both as researchers and as physicians. Such an expectation, it might be maintained, creates psychological tensions in the mind of the physicians because they are being required to play two very different roles at one and the same time. More realistically, the argument continues, some sort of independent review body should be used which would withhold the scientific information from the physician and decide when the RCT should be concluded.

Now this solution has the merit of removing the tension from the mind of the experimenters, but the ethical dilemma remains as it was before. The important ethical issue is whether and when it is ethically permissible to carry out the trials and what the justification for them is said to be, rather than the procedural question of who knows what.

We have looked at only one of the attempts to deny the reality of the dilemma but would wish to argue that no method of avoiding it is really satisfactory. It seems preferable to admit the reality of the dilemma and to concede that there must be some kind of a trade-off between the ethical requirements to advance therapeutic knowledge for the future and to give the best known treatment for given patients at a given time. Harm to patients cannot of course entirely be prevented by local research ethics committees, even after the most detailed scrutiny of research proposals; what the committees can do is to ensure that adequate information is provided and consent obtained and thus prevent harms being turned into wrongs.

11.3 Local research ethics committees

Local research ethics committees (LRECs) were officially established in the UK in the early 1990s although they had existed in a more haphazard form for many years before then. They were set up to give ethical advice on research proposals, and although in the UK their advice is restricted to NHS bodies, it is not likely that research would be published by any journal of repute unless it had received ethical approval. Research ethics committees have been in existence for longer in the US.

It is recommended that an LREC should have 8–12 members. This should allow for a sufficiently broad range of experience and expertise, so that the scientific and medical aspects of a research proposal can be reconciled with the welfare of research subjects, and broader ethical implications (Royal College of Physicians 1990; Department of Health 1991).

Members should be drawn from both sexes and from a wide age range. They should include:

- hospital medical and appropriate scientific staff
- nursing staff
- general practitioners
- two or more lay persons.

Although drawn from groups identified with particular interests or responsibilities in connection with health issues, LREC members do not represent those groups. They are appointed in their own right, to participate in the work of the LREC as individuals of sound judgement and relevant experience.

The considerations which ought to weigh with the committee are listed. The LREC will need to know:

(i)   Has the scientific merit of the proposal been (or will it be) properly assessed?

(ii)   How will the health of the research subjects be affected?

(iii) Are there possible hazards and, if so, adequate facilities to deal with them?

(iv)   What degree of discomfort or distress is foreseen?

(v)   Is the investigation adequately supervised and is the supervisor responsible for the project adequately qualified and experienced?

(vi)   What monetary or other inducements are being offered to the NHS body, doctors, researchers, subjects, or anyone else involved?

(vii) Are there proper procedures for providing explanation and for obtaining consent from the subjects or, where necessary, their parents or guardians?

(viii) Has the appropriate information sheet for the subjects been prepared?

The document makes it clear that *all* research using human subjects, whether therapeutic or non-therapeutic, must be submitted for approval.

11.4 Consent

LRECs can advise research bodies, but in the end the only solution to the ethical dilemmas of medical research can come from the voluntary consent of the subjects involved. Only if patients or research subjects are willing to say 'I waive my right to the best known therapy' or 'I voluntarily agree to be a subject for the investigation which has been outlined to me' is there any ethical legitimacy for research on human subjects. Indeed, as we shall see, problems still remain in the palliative area. But let us first look briefly at consent. The document (Department of Health 1991) says the following on consent:

The procedure for obtaining consent will vary according to the nature of each research proposal. The LREC will want to be satisfied on the level and amount of information to be given to a prospective subject. Some methods of study such as randomised controlled trials need to be explained to subjects with particular care to ensure that valid consent is obtained. The LREC will want to look at such proposals particularly carefully. They will also want to check that all subjects are told that they are free to withdraw without explanation or hindrance at any stage of the procedure and with no detriment to their treatment. An information sheet, to be kept by the subject, should be required in almost all cases.

Written consent should be required for all research, except where the most trivial of procedures is concerned. For therapeutic research consent should be recorded in the patient's medical records.

Some research proposals will draw their subjects from groups of people who may find it difficult or impossible to give their consent, for example the unconscious, the very elderly, the mentally disordered or some other vulnerable group. In considering these proposals the LREC should seek

appropriate specialist advice and they will need to examine the proposal
with particular care to satisfy themselves that proceeding without valid
consent is ethically acceptable.

11.5   Special ethical problems of research in palliative care

The existence of LRECs certainly has improved the ethical quality of
research, even if only to remind researchers that research has an
ethical dimension. But serious problems remain, especially in the
area of palliative medicine. We shall now consider what these are,
and concentrate in the first instance on autonomous patients.

The first special problem in palliative research is that the patients
concerned may be in pain or discomfort, distressed or frightened.
As a result of this they will be more vulnerable than other patients
and more dependent on their carers. This raises the question as to
whether they can ever give consent which is truly voluntary. Patients
in non-terminal settings are sometimes said to feel constrained and
bound to consent to a request to take part in a research study; if
so then patients who are in a terminal state may all the more feel
constrained.

Secondly, it might be argued that patients in a terminal state, by
the nature of their situation, have limited time left and should be left
in peace to share such time with their friends and relatives without
having new treatments tried out on them. Of course some patients
are anxious either to contribute to medical knowledge or to try any
new therapeutic options that may be available in trials. Connected
with the second argument there is a third: when patients are in a
terminal condition they are likely to be closer to their relatives and
friends than at any other time, and it is likely that the relatives will
feel distress if they think that new therapies are being tried out at this
ultimate period in the relationship. Do these considerations suggest
research in the field of terminal care cannot be ethically justified?
Not necessarily. We should perhaps first review some of the types of
research which are possible in this area, for research is by no means
all of the same sort and different sorts raise different issues.

The first category of possible research in the palliative field we
might term epidemiological research, by which we mean research
based on a study of a variety of records. For example, there are
studies of the survival times of patients with tumours of different
sorts and with different age and sex distribution. Again, there could

be research into the distribution of diseases, and their correlation with various types of lifestyle.

Secondly, there could be research reviewing people's preferences for dying at home, in hospital, or in a hospice, and assessing the kinds and quality of care available in these settings. Research of this general sort does not seem to raise serious ethical problems, although access to records always requires assurances about confidentiality.

A third sort of 'research' which does not raise serious, if any, ethical problems is therapeutic research based on the doctor's own experience, sometimes called 'innovative therapy'. Indeed, some would argue that this does not constitute research (Royal College of Physicians 1990). For the benefit of a particular patient, and with that patient's consent, the doctor uses a treatment in a novel or non-standard way. For example, a doctor may find after some years of prescribing a certain treatment that it is possible to reach some provisional generalizations—say, that in his or her experience certain drugs or combinations of drugs are especially effective for certain purposes. That doctor applies that knowledge for the benefit of a particular patient. The scientific purist may criticize such historically based research as anecdotal and not significant. None the less, a great deal of medical knowledge develops in just that way. If an experiment in the context of innovative therapy proves successful, then true research must be carried out to evaluate the treatment before it is recommended for wider use. It may be regrettable, but the practice of medicine is influenced less by the reading of research papers than by observation and experience in clinical situations. Moreover, medical education at the clinical level is largely education by apprenticeship and this process of 'see one, do one, teach one' is as influential in the accumulation of medical knowledge as reading the research paper. The ethical problems raised by this kind of experience-based research are those of consent to *treatment* rather than consent to *research*.

A fourth sort of research does raise ethical problems, and that is research based on interviews with the patient or the relatives. It is worth stressing that such research does raise ethical problems because it is easy to fall into the trap of thinking that only invasive or drug-related care raises serious ethical problems. But an interview which involves painful questions, or even a questionnaire, can be just as distressing. This may be especially the case if the study is directed at some sort of evaluation of the care being received. For example, if a study were to involve questioning relatives or patients about the nature and extent of the information supplied by the team on the disease, this could cause distress. This is a serious matter at any state but a scrutiny of the doctor–patient or nurse–patient relationship at the end of life is especially difficult and requires to be handled with great sensitivity. On the other hand, some kind of audit of care is necessary in the palliative field as well as in other fields of health care.

Finally, we must look at the use of RCTs in palliative care. McWhinney *et al.* (1994) describe the failure of an RCT designed to evaluate a palliative care home support team based on an in-patient unit. Patients in the study group received the service immediately, while those in the control group received it after one month. The main comparison point was at one month. Pain and nausea levels were measured at entry to the trial and at one month. The quality of life of the patients and the care-givers was also measured.

The RCT failed, and the authors provide a number of interesting reasons for the failure. There were early deaths, problems of recruitment to the study, and a low compliance rate for completion of questionnaires. The factors bringing about the failure are not hard to explain. Death is obviously likely to be a frequent occurrence in the palliative area when the trial lasts one month. Moreover, it will obviously be difficult to obtain completed questionnaires from weak and sick patients, and carers, knowing this, will be reluctant to cooperate in studies and may discourage recruitment to trials. The authors conclude that RCTs may prove to be impracticable in the palliative care service, and they are fully aware of the ethical problems of attempting such trials with very sick or dying patients.

In the same volume of the *British Medical Journal* McQuay and Moore (1994) attempt to defend the employment of RCTs in palliative care research. They are clear that RCTs are the 'gold standard' in medical research, and wonder, in a sinister way, whether medical decisions not supported by RCTs will continue to be purchased. They agree that while it may not be ethically wrong to use patients on a waiting list as controls if they have stable chronic conditions, it is hard to find ethical justification for randomization to treatment versus delayed treatment in the palliative care area. But they deny that it follows that all RCTs must be ruled out from the ethical standpoint in palliative care. They suggest that 'comparison of two interventions, neither of which is known to be superior, would be the classic equipoise requirement for ethical randomization'.

What seems to emerge from an examination of these two points of view is that it may be possible to devise RCTs for palliative care which can satisfy the *ethical* criteria we have been using in this book. This conclusion, however, does not meet all the practical difficulties of recruitment, compliance, and completion, especially in view of the known reluctance of professionals in palliative care to encourage their patients to participate.

So far we have been discussing research on subjects competent to give consent—autonomous subjects. What of the non-autonomous who, through physical or mental incapacity, are not competent to consent? According to the Law Commission (1995) *Report on mental incapacity* 6.29: 'non-therapeutic research on patients who do not have capacity to consent is illegal and amounts to an unlawful battery'. It is often thought by funding bodies and ethics committees that consent by a relative will validate research on such subjects, but the Law Commission Report states that 'As a matter of law, such "consent" is meaningless'.

Nevertheless, there is a case for saying that such research should be made legal with stringent safeguards. It may be permissible to conduct therapeutic research on the non-autonomous patient, provided the safeguards mentioned in the Declaration of Helsinki (II 2) are observed—'The potential benefits, hazards and discomforts of a new method should be weighed against the advantages of the best current diagnostic and therapeutic methods'. The Declaration of Helsinki is here referring to therapeutic research, but it is harder to find ethical justification for non-therapeutic research on the non-autonomous patient. There is a difference here between the non-autonomous patient in palliative care and children or the mentally handicapped. Children and the mentally handicapped may not be legally competent to give consent but to a greater or lesser extent the nature of what is proposed can be explained to them. But with the non-autonomous patient in palliative care this may not be possible because of their disease state. Nevertheless, it is still possible to make out a case for non-therapeutic research on non-autonomous subjects provided certain conditions are satisfied. These conditions are very helpfully stated by the Law Commission. First, they recommend that there should be a statutory committee to be known as the Mental Incapacity Research Committee, by which non-therapeutic research proposals should be reviewed. Our only reservation on this is the difficulty of persuading people to participate in yet another committee! Perhaps special meetings of existing research committees with additional coopted members would suffice.

The second proposal of the Law Commission (6.34) is that committees may approve proposed research if satisfied:

(1)   that it is desirable to provide knowledge of the causes or treatment of, or of the care of people affected by, the incapacitating condition with which any participant is or may be affected,

(2)   that the object of the research cannot be effectively achieved without the participation of persons who are or may be without capacity to consent, and

(3)   that the research will not expose a participant to more than negligible risk, will not be unduly invasive or restrictive of a participant and will not unduly interfere with a participant's freedom of action or privacy.

In reviewing research proposals research committees are normally concerned simply with protocols, the assumption being that the subjects of research, in so far as they are able to consent, are all ethically eligible. But the Law Commission points out (6.36) that in the case of the non-autonomous subject this assumption is not valid and there is therefore 'a need for a separate and individualised independent check to confirm whether a particular proposed participant should indeed by brought into the project'. In other words the recommendation for research on non-autonomous subjects requires a two-tier process. In addition to the scrutiny of protocols already recommended as above, there is a third recommendation that non-therapeutic research in relation to a person without capacity should require either:

(1)   court approval,

(2)   the consent of an attorney or manager,

(3)   a certificate from a doctor not involved in the research that the participation of the person is appropriate, or

(4)   designation of the research as not involving direct contact.

Since in the context of palliative care many patients will be in a non-autonomous condition for a period, especially just prior to death, research would be helpful in yielding information about the possible benefits, risks, and harms of treatments which could be used at this stage. For example, there is debate about whether artificial hydration would alleviate distress in patients with diminished consciousness prior to death, whilst there is coexistent anxiety that it might increase pulmonary secretions or perhaps prolong the dying process. However, research in this area would entail research on non-autonomous patients who could not consent contemporaneously to take part (although one could argue that they might be able to consent in advance). Such research would entail randomizing patients into two groups, one to receive artificial hydration and one not, and then assessing their distress and subsequent events. Invasive procedures such as blood tests would provide helpful information. Research projects like this are fraught with moral problems because the patients are unable to consent, are unlikely themselves to benefit from the research, and will be subjected to blood tests. Yet without such research the balance of benefits to harms and risks of artificial hydration in this situation cannot be determined. The only reasonable solution seems to be that necessary research projects on non-autonomous patients are very tightly regulated, as has been suggested above.

11.6 Conclusions

1. Any kind of research involving human subjects is likely to raise ethical problems, but research in the palliative field is especially sensitive.

2. Randomized clinical trials create the most ethical problems, but they are not the only research method.

3. Local research committee approval confers some measure of legitimacy on research.

4. But the consent of the participants is the key issue and must be handled with extreme care in palliative medicine.

5. It may be possible to design randomized clinical trials which meet the ethical problems in palliative care but practical difficulties of recruitment, compliance, and completion are likely to remain.

6. Research on the non-autonomous patient is fraught with ethical difficulties, but it may be ethically permissible provided stringent safeguards are met.

12
Resource allocation

Annual income twenty pounds, annual expenditure nineteen nineteen six, result happiness.
Annual income twenty pounds, annual expenditure twenty pounds ought and six, result misery.
                Charles Dickens, *David Copperfield*, Ch. 12
                (Mr Micawber) (1805)

Good health is a state which all people desire, and which is regarded as important for human flourishing. There is a moral imperative to gain maximum benefits from health care resources and to distribute those benefits justly. Ironically, health care cannot guarantee health, and the function of palliative care is not to restore health but to minimize the adverse impact of disease and death on human flourishing.

The process of resource allocation comprises two separate functions. Macroallocation is the process of deciding how much money should be spent and how it will be obtained, what kind of services should be available and to which population, who will provide the services, and how the power to control them will be distributed. Microallocation is the process of deciding which individuals from the population requiring the service should actually receive it, assuming that the available supply of services is limited by resource constraints and that need and/or demand exceed supply.

12.1 The concept of need in palliative care

The concept of need is crucial to the moral issues arising in both macro- and microallocation of resources, but it is complex and problematic. Usually the term 'need' describes a necessary condition for the attainment of some end-state. For example, nurses need a certain level of knowledge to pass their final examinations, people need clothes and fuel and food to keep warm, and so on: the need is related to some end-state. What is the end-state for palliative care 'needs'? Egalitarians might say that palliative care is needed (and therefore should be resourced and distributed) so as to restore all those with a terminal illness to the same acceptable level of well-being for their remaining lives, but even maximum specialist palliative care cannot restore all patients to the *same* level because illnesses and human reactions to them are so variable. The aim of palliative care is not therefore to enable all patients to exist in an equal state of well-being. Rather it is to minimize the adverse effects of illness and death on each individual patient and family. Specific goals such as pain and symptom control exist, but even the best care cannot grant complete physical comfort and some symptoms such as fatigue will persist. Nor can palliative care guarantee psychosocial and spiritual well-being. Therefore there is no universal and specific end-state or outcome which palliative care is aiming to achieve and by which its success may be judged.

The absence of this end-state makes assessment of need difficult, and problems in allocating resources on the basis of need then logically follow. The problem of need in palliative care has to be approached from another direction. Beauchamp and Childress (1994) have suggested that a need is 'something without which one will be fundamentally harmed'. This is helpful, at least if it refers to basic needs, in that it stresses that the harm resulting must be 'fundamental' and not simply trivial. We might say that this means that the existence of the person must be threatened or perhaps that their ability to function as a human being is seriously impaired.

There are two comments which must be made on this simple but useful description of need. The first is that one still has to decide what in practice constitutes a fundamental harm, and this is no easy matter. For example, pain is almost universally regarded as a fundamental harm because it seriously impairs ability to function and flourish, but in the context of palliative care death is not ultimately regarded as a harm, but as the inevitable conclusion of life. The second comment is that it is the human condition including the illness and mortality which causes harm to occur. Therefore it might be preferable to say that a health care need is something without the satisfaction of which one will come to fundamental harm.

Fundamental harm may be described as a state contrary to the most important interests of the human being. A need is then 'something without which one will come to be in a state which is contrary to one's most important interests'. This is a more acceptable and appropriate description of the meaning of the term 'need' in the context of palliative care because it emphasizes that the desirable state is relative to the circumstances in which one finds oneself. 'Interests' is a better term than 'harms', because there are few specific harms, apart perhaps from physical distress, that appear to be universal.

Interests are both subjective and objective; rational people are capable of determining their own self-interests, although others may disagree on the basis of objective criteria of best interests. For instance, a patient with a breast cancer may decline surgery in the belief that, for her, an operation or a lumpectomy scar is worse than either the possibility of a fungating mass or death. She may decline operation for rational reasons which accord with her self-interests, but others would say that lumpectomy was in her 'best' interests and that therefore she 'needed' the operation. This example illustrates that interests can be subjective and objective. It follows that needs can be subjective and objective. Needs are subjective if one is talking about one's perceived self-interests, or objective if the interests are as seen by others.

Disparity may occur between subjective and objective interests and therefore between subjective and objective ideas of needs. A middle-aged man dying of lung cancer was seen living in a garden shed in a wet field. When offered a hospital bed he initially declined, saying he was sure that others needed it more than he did. It was difficult for the carers to imagine a patient more in need than he was. His concept of need was different from theirs!

Wants or demands must also be distinguished from needs. People are able to differentiate between those things which they would simply like or desire, and those without which they would be in a state which they consider fundamentally harmful because it is contrary to their most important interests. For example, patients may want a specialist nurse to talk to about feelings with regard to a terminal illness, but they may simultaneously acknowledge that they have trusted friends, a general practitioner, and a community nurse to whom they could also confide. In this situation they want but do not need the specialist nurse. On the other hand, a very isolated individual might both want and be in need of such specialist help. Whether a particular patient needs specialist palliative care input in addition to competent and compassionate general health care depends on many factors, including the complexity and difficulty of symptom control and emotional and social factors.

This leads us to the conclusion that patients cannot be said to 'need' everything which they and others consider they could benefit from. This distinction is important, because health care is quite rightly resourced according to need for the good reason that members of society cannot be expected to fund from taxation everything that patients could benefit from. A health or palliative care need is not simply 'something one would benefit from having'. If this were so, expectations of health care would be infinite, and could not possibly ever be reconciled to finite resources. For example, patients with terminal illnesses might all benefit from specialist palliative care, or even luxury holidays, but one could not say that *all* patients need either of these resources.

So far we have discussed need as it relates to the individual, but the concept has important social consequences because in health care it seems generally to imply an 'ought' or duty on behalf of society to meet those needs. Thus if patients can be said to need certain palliative care services in order to minimize suffering, then society has a duty to provide those services if it is committed to the relief of that suffering. This sense of obligation or duty may arise from the social application of the principle of beneficence (one ought to help those in need), or perhaps from justice (everyone ought to have equal opportunities to flourish by minimizing illness-related suffering), or perhaps from a community desire to sustain and emphasize the intrinsic worth of each of its members by providing for their needs even in terminal illness when they can no longer be materially productive. This association between need and the 'ought' to meet it is so strong that health care planners may be reluctant to identify a need or admit the extent of it because acknowledgement of its existence implies a duty to supply resources. The concept of need has also become entangled with the idea that each individual has a *right* to the palliative care services required to meet their needs. In fact it is difficult to argue that sick individuals have an absolute right to demand that others in the community should pay for their health care.

For example, whilst citizens of affluent countries with health services may consider palliative care a right, citizens of impoverished countries have no such rights because they cannot impose an 'ought' on the poor communities to provide services which they simply cannot afford. This illustrates the fact that people cannot have a right to palliative care, and impose a moral 'ought' on others to provide it, when that moral ought is impossible to carry out.

12.2 Macroallocation of resources

12.2.1 *Community responsibility for the provision of palliative care*

Most Western societies consider that there is a strong moral obligation to provide at least a decent minimum level of palliative care. There are several reasons for this moral imperative. It is probably based on community ideas of beneficence (doing good and minimizing harm) and also on ideas of justice in relation to equal opportunity. Suffering due to disease seems to be distributed randomly, almost like a natural lottery, and palliative care is one way to minimize the inequality of suffering. Good palliative care is also seen as a social insurance policy—community members are willing to contribute in order to ensure that services will exist for themselves and their families when they need them. Finally, the moral imperative to provide care for the dying may be based on a perceived need to sustain and emphasize the worth of all community members. A commitment to palliative care demonstrates that the community places a value on the welfare of each individual which is not dependent on material productivity.

The resulting moral obligation to provide a decent minimum of palliative care is so strong that it is often socially enforced; services are funded at least in part through taxation, and voluntary giving to charitable sources of care is also encouraged. Two further questions essential to resource allocation follow: first, what constitutes that decent minimum level of care, and secondly, is there a moral obligation to provide more than the minimum level of care?

Standards describing a decent minimum level of care are being produced, and relate both to the sort of services to be provided and the quality of those services. It is now generally agreed that all health care workers should be competent in giving information and basic symptom control, and should have awareness of the importance of listening to patients' psychosocial and spiritual problems and addressing these where possible. All professional carers should have the appropriate attitudes of dedication to the patient's total good (beneficence) and of respect for autonomy. It is also agreed that access to specialist services is required for those patients with difficult or complex problems. It seems likely that palliative care services will continue to develop in affluent societies until this minimum level of care is available to all, and it now seems morally unacceptable for an affluent society to fail to fund a decent minimum level of palliative care from central sources.

The degree of moral obligation to provide more than this minimum level of care is more problematic. Difficulties arise when individuals or the community as a whole feel that they ought to provide palliative care at more than a minimum level but cannot adequately resource that extra care. It is then necessary to limit the scope of care available to all, and/or to be selective about who receives it, and/or to raise extra funds from charitable sources. We have already stated that resources are necessarily limited, and that there cannot be a moral 'ought' to provide unlimited palliative care precisely because this is impossible from limited resources. More-over, the general duty of beneficence is not unlimited so there is no duty to provide unlimited palliative care. Therefore, whilst there is a strong obligation to provide for patients' basic palliative care needs, there is no moral obligation to provide everything that those terminally ill could benefit from. There may be a weak obligation to provide as much care over and above the minimum level the society can reasonably afford, and there does seem to be moral justification for raising charitable funds to supplement minimum care.

It is sometimes assumed that society has a duty to strive to the utmost to alleviate all the effects of terminal illness, and it is implied that if it fails to do so then it is causally responsible for them. This is surely not the case. When a person suffers distress as a result of terminal illness, society is not causally responsible for it. The society may be held morally responsible for failing to alleviate the suffering only if it could have been prevented by the application of a decent minimum level of care which the society can resource and has undertaken as a community to provide. For example, an affluent society with a centrally funded national health service would be blameworthy if it failed to provide adequate basic pain control to a patient who therefore suffered pain which could have been alleviated by provision of a basic level of medications, knowledge, and skill. Such a society should be held blameworthy for this omission, just as it would be held blameworthy for the suffering and death of a diabetic patient who died as a result of failure to provide a basic and adequate insulin regime to control the patient's diabetes.

Most health care professionals are not involved in deciding the size of the health care budget nor how much of it should be spent on specialist palliative care. None the less, they should do their utmost to inform planners of the services required to provide a decent minimum level of care, so as to ensure that it is available to *all*. When this has been achieved, and in justice it seems fair to say *only* when this has been achieved, should debate then turn to providing more than basic care.

12.2.2   *Charitable provision of care*

Historically, there has been a gap between statutory health care service provision in the area of palliative care and that which is necessary to meet even basic needs. This gap is partly financial, but is also partly educational in that not all health care workers have the necessary knowledge base and skills. Many charities have tried to fill both the financial and educational gap, and have achieved a great deal in so doing.

In the United Kingdom palliative care services have developed largely through the activity of charities and consequently there has been no needs assessment or central planning. As a result, services tend to be patchy and some areas have no specialist service, whereas others may have several specialist centres providing much more than basic care and aiming to supply every amenity from which the patient could benefit. The level of palliative care expertise in the sphere of general health care is also very variable. There is therefore great inequality of palliative care provision.

Some patients benefit from specialist care in a luxury environment provided by local charities, whereas others receive less than adequate care. At first sight this situation seems morally unacceptable but there are good moral reasons for allowing charitable provision of care. For example, it can be argued that a community must be entitled to fund a superior service from charitable sources for its own members if it so chooses. It is also important to preserve the principles that money given for a particular purpose should be used to that end, and that people should be completely free to give to whatever charity they choose. In fact it is not the provision of more than basic care by charities which is unacceptable, but rather the absence of a universally available decent minimum level of care which is unacceptable. This latter problem can be solved only by planning and resourcing services centrally, so that they form an integrated network through which all patients have access to the care which they need.

Having said this there are some moral issues which arise with regard to the raising of charitable funds to provide palliative care. Charities should be honest about the true need for the services they provide. For example, if a luxury environment and high staffing levels are to be available, this should be publicized so that people can choose whether to donate funds to this end. Moreover, the need which the charity purports to meet should be clearly established; this is because declaring something to be a health care need is associated with a moral 'ought' that individuals should contribute to it. Therefore, if emotive advertising is used to fund-raise for a 'need', the public will be under some moral pressure to subscribe to it. One must question whether money is being raised to meet true needs, that is to provide essential services, or if it is being raised simply because some people consider those services essential. It is of course justifiable to fund-raise on the basis of enhancing services so as to meet more than basic needs, and this should be explicit in fund-raising publicity.

Money raised from voluntary donation should be used to maximum benefit. Administrators of charitable funds have a responsibility to make the best use of funds which they hold in trust. This may cause conflicts between ideas of distributive justice and the aims of the charity. For example, a charity may want to fund a high-profile centre of excellence which will attract publicity and therefore future donations, whereas a less conspicuous but much needed basic service could be provided to a larger number of patients in an area with little existing service. The principles of distributive justice may in this case suggest the latter course of action, but the charity may have a vested interest in pursuing the former course. Complex and difficult moral decisions of this nature are made constantly by the administrators of charitable funds.

12.2.3 *Specialist versus general palliative care*

All patients with an illness which is terminal require care which is by definition palliative, and where the predominant focus is improved quality of life. The needs of most patients can be met by health care workers who are not specialists in palliative care but who possess appropriate knowledge and skills and approach patients with morally appropriate attitudes. Whilst the majority of patients would benefit from specialist services, whether as in-patients, day-patients, or in the domiciliary setting, not all patients actually need those specialist services in that they will not sustain serious impediment to their interests by not receiving them.

Nevertheless, it is acknowledged that some patients do have complex and difficult problems which may be solved only by using the specialist knowledge and skills of those who work constantly in palliative care. The likelihood of meeting the needs of this group of patients is far greater if they obtain help from a specialist team, either at home or in specialist facilities. There seems to be a *strong* moral obligation to provide adequate specialist palliative care to meet the needs of this group of patients, and central health care funds should be used to this end. This should be considered as part of the decent minimum level of palliative care because the needs of these patients can be met only by the application of specialist knowledge and skills.

There is a *weak* moral obligation to provide specialist care to those who would benefit from it but whose basic needs could be met through the statutory services. Since health care resources will always be limited, it is unlikely that central community funding will be available to provide specialist care for these patients, and it seems legitimate to use charitable funding to this end.

A just distribution of specialist resources is morally required, as is education for all health care workers regarding palliative care; to ensure these ends are achieved central planning is essential. If specialist services or education are purchased from the voluntary sector, control over the nature and standard of the service is exercised via a contract. Unfortunately, moral problems occur with this arrangement because the charitable organization may be reliant on the contract for revenue, and may be forced by that reliance to try to meet inappropriate or unrealistic performance targets set by purchasers.

Ultimately, all power over provision of palliative care services lies with the purchasers of that care, since they hold the budget and negotiate all contracts over which they have an effective monopoly. This seems unsatisfactory, because unless the purchaser is a person of great integrity who understands the nature and aims of palliative care, the services provided will be less than optimal. It is unfortunate that this power to plan and implement services is not more widely distributed—if it were, a more just process of decision making would be more likely.

12.2.4 *Economic analysis*

Palliative care services have developed in response to need, but planning and resource allocation of health care in general is increasingly subject to economic analysis. This analysis is appropriate because it constitutes one aspect of attempts to obtain maximum benefit from the use of resources according to the principle of utility (the duty to seek the greatest happiness of the greatest number). It is also necessary for attempts to distribute those benefits of health care justly. Economic analysis is only one morally relevant item in health care planning and resource allocation. Important moral principles such as respect for autonomy and individual choice, the social obligations of doing good and preventing or removing harms, and the claims of justice, fairness, or equality are all relevant and important in health care planning and therefore in the allocation of resources to palliative care.

Unfortunately, economic analysis in palliative care is extremely difficult because it entails ascribing financial values to many aspects of palliative care, some of which can be measured in monetary terms and some of which simply cannot. The current economic language of resource allocation is that of 'costs and benefits'. The aim is to achieve the maximum benefit for a given cost, and to distribute that benefit justly.

Costs and benefits can be assessed both qualitatively (in terms of their nature) and quantitatively (in terms of money or other unit of measurement). Costs and benefits arise at all stages of the delivery of palliative care. These stages comprise input, process, output, and outcome. Inputs are resources of money, buildings and technology, and human effort. The process is what health care workers actually do, and necessarily entails some benefits related to the way patients perceive they are cared for. Indeed much of the benefit of palliative care is attributable to the process itself, especially in the sphere of emotional care. Outputs are the characteristics of the service, such

as symptom control, practical nursing care, emotional support,
rehabilitation, and so on. Outcome is the effect on the patient,
family, and community as the end result of the palliative care provided over a period of time for the patient. Outcome is judged
objectively and subjectively by the patient, by the community, and by
the professional staff involved. It must be related to the objectives of
care set by the patient and staff at the start of the episode of care.
Outputs and outcomes entail objective measures where possible, but
also subjective evaluation and value judgements. The community
should be involved in assessing outcome since this is an important
factor in resource allocation.

We have distinguished outputs and outcome to emphasize that the
latter is the *overall effect* of palliative care, and comprises effects on
the quality of life and indeed the quality of death of the patient,
effects on the experience of the family and their bereavement, and
effects on the community.

It is obvious that it is not possible to ascribe numerical values to
many of the outputs of palliative care, nor to the outcomes. Whilst
patients can estimate, say on a scale of 1 to 10, how good care was,
they cannot meaningfully describe the value of that care to themselves in numerical terms. It is also extremely difficult to attribute
perceived changes of quality of life or death to the care provided,
since the effects of care cannot be isolated from other influences such
as family and social support or the variable course of illness. It is
therefore difficult to assess the outputs and outcome of palliative
care in numerical terms. It is also arguably impossible to put a
financial value on the outputs and outcomes of palliative care. Any
scale of financial value devised is likely to be invalid and unreliable
and therefore useless for the purposes of economic analysis of the
benefits of care. Similarly, the costs in human terms of the input and
process of care cannot be expressed in financial terms, and thus
analysis of costs is limited to financial aspects only.

Thus economic analysis of the costs and benefits of palliative
care is very limited, and it is important that this is acknowledged
in resource allocation. Economists wish to assess the nature and
magnitude of costs and benefits, so as to weigh them in some sort
of balance. It has to be said that it is difficult to weigh in any sort
of balance items which are 'different sorts of thing' and are therefore incommensurable. We cannot apply a reasonably valid and
reliable numerical scale to many of the factors in the input–process–

output–outcome balance, and so we cannot assess and compare those factors in numerical terms at all. Some benefits cannot be quantified.

Attempts have been made to describe and compare different health care benefits in numerical terms, combining quality and quantity of life gained in a single measure such as the quality-adjusted life-year or QALY. There are many moral and practical problems in the derivation and use of the QALY, but they are not relevant to this discussion because the QALY is simply not applicable to palliative care—in the QALY numerical scale death is rated at 0 and health at 1, so at the conclusion of palliative care when the patient has died an inevitable score of 0 for the outcome of the episode would be gained. In palliative care extension of life is not the main objective and it is not possible to know if care influenced the length of life. Moreover, the impact of care on quality of life is difficult to assess and express in numerical terms.

It is therefore not possible to compare in financial terms the benefits of palliative care per unit cost with the benefits per unit cost of other interventions such as hip replacements and coronary bypasses. Even if it were, difficult moral decisions would remain, because financial considerations comprise only one of the morally relevant factors in the decisions which society has to make concerning allocation of health care resources.

What we can derive is a simple cost-effectiveness analysis where financial costs are compared with the effects of care such as symptom control, practical care, relief of anxiety for patient and family, good communication of information, and reduced mortality and morbidity in bereavement. The financial costs of achieving the benefits of palliative care by different methods can be compared. This does not mean that each benefit actually has a true value in monetary terms, any more than a life has a value in monetary terms. It is not true that something is 'always worth what people are willing to pay for it' because the value of some things, such as human beings, love, and works of art cannot be equated with money. It is a gross oversimplification to express the value of the benefits of palliative care simply in terms of money.

Ultimately, society has to decide how much money should be allocated to achieve the benefits of a decent minimum level of care for all. Whilst some of that funding will be needed for specialist palliative care services, it is morally obligatory to devote some funds to the education of health care workers so that they have the knowledge and skill base necessary for competence.

12.3 Microallocation of resources

Specialist palliative care cannot be provided for everyone who would benefit from it. It is likely that for the foreseeable future it may not be available even for all those who need it—those who without it are very likely to sustain avoidable fundamental harm. Ideally, society should decide what level of care should be provided and that care should be made equally available to all. Unfortunately, this is often not the case and therefore doctors, nurses, and social workers must decide which patients will receive the help they need, and which will not.

In-patient beds, day-centre places, and access to specialist nurses are all finite resources which cannot ultimately be 'shared' by ever-increasing numbers of patients. Morally justifiable grounds for discriminating between patients have to be established and used. This process is commonly described as rationing. It is important that the process of rationing at the individual patient level should in itself be just, as far as possible. No process can guarantee the most desirable outcome in each rationing instance because the disease outcome for each patient is so uncertain, but it is essential that the process itself is just.

The requirements of distributive justice would seem to indicate that as many patients as possible should be given adequate care from the resources available. This may not strictly equate with deriving the maximum benefit from those resources, but it does accord with ideas of fairness which moderate the use of the principle of utility. Some patients may receive more than adequate care, but it seems that this is not morally justifiable if it occurs at the cost of denying adequate care to others.

There are different ideas about what criteria for distinguishing or discriminating between patients are morally just. Rationing systems rely on these selection criteria. Distinguishing between patients is not in itself morally wrong—indeed it is morally required whenever rationing is unavoidable. What is important is that distinctions should not be made between patients who are actually similar in relevant respects, and distinctions should be made between patients who are actually different in relevant respects.

Several ways of discriminating between patients for the purposes of rationing palliative care are used and seem morally justifiable. Reference to common clinical scenarios helps to clarify the moral issues.

Initially, a decision is made about which patient population is eligible for the service. This decision should be made with public consultation, assuming that the public are resourcing the service. Historically, specialist palliative care services were available to patients with cancer or motor neurone disease, but now political consultation and public demand has resulted in all patients with a terminal illness being considered eligible for the services. This is likely to result in a much greater demand which will far outstrip supply, and stringent selection criteria will be essential to allow a just process of rationing. Patients who live outside the catchment area may be refused care on the grounds that the primary duty of the service is to local residents. This policy would limit patient choice. On the other hand, such patients may be accepted in preference to local patients if financial resources for their care accompany them. It would not seem just to deny access to local patients because financial advantages accompanied those from outside the catchment area.

The most common criterion for patient selection is called *medical utility*. This is basically the differential value of the treatment for different patients (or how much the patients can benefit) and as such it is obviously a value judgement. The principle is that the resources should be used to maximize the welfare of patients in need of treatment. Medical utility has to do with both patient need for the specialist palliative care service and also with the prospects of the desired outcome or success from that service.

Patient need is not an easy criterion to use for selection because patients have many different sorts of need which are not comparable. Different sorts of thing are inclined to be incommensurable. For instance, one patient might need admission for symptom control to relieve a difficult neurogenic pain which has not responded to treatment at home, another might need 24-hour care, emotional support and rehabilitation because of paraplegia, a young AIDS patient may need respite care to give his exhausted family a break, and yet another may be dying, in need of medical and nursing care and accompanied by emotionally and physically exhausted relatives.

These needs are all genuine, but because they are different we cannot weigh them in a balance against each other. Therefore we tend to look at other criteria we consider relevant in order to decide which patient should receive the specialist service.

In many areas of health care such as coronary bypass surgery and resuscitation on an intensive care unit, the *likelihood of success* of treatment is used as a selection criterion. This is justifiable since it is wrong to give treatment to patients in whom it is unlikely to succeed in preference to those with a good chance of a successful outcome such as survival.

The moral situation in palliative care is much more complex. First, one must consider how success in terms of outcome is assessed. We have said that overall improvement in quality of life and death is the important outcome measure for the patient. Quality in this sense is composed of many factors, including psychosocial aspects of well-being as well physical comfort. There are multiple end-points of care, many of which are not numerically quantifiable and all of which are difficult to assess. Moreover, standards of success are relative to what may reasonably be expected for each aspect of distress. It is complex and difficult in the clinical context to assess success in terms of outcome, and therefore moral problems arise in using the likelihood of success as a selection criterion for specialist care.

For example, choosing which patient to admit for pain control based on the likelihood of success is a complex practical and moral issue. Standards of success for each cause of pain are relative to reasonable expectations in the light of knowledge and experience. Neurogenic pain is notoriously difficult to relieve completely, side-effects of treatment are likely, and the patient may be left with some distress resulting from paraesthesiae (a sensation of 'pins and needles'). Therefore our standard will not be complete relief of pain with restoration of normal sensation because this is unrealistic. Instead we would consider success to be substantial relief of pain, with reduced overall distress which is bearable to the patient. Standards of success in terms of outcome should also be established by patients. Those with neurogenic pain might consider a regime satisfactory if it reduces distress with minimal side-effects and risks, even if it gives incomplete relief of pain. In contrast, metastatic bone pain is easier to relieve using multiple therapeutic approaches, and complete pain relief at rest would be considered a reasonable

standard of success. It is more likely that we can achie
plete relief at rest than that we can achieve even partia
many neurogenic pains. Does this mean we should give res
preferentially to patients with bone pain, assuming other relev
factors such as patient distress are roughly equal? This conclusion
seems intuitively wrong, and so further consideration is needed.

It is possible that in palliative care the likelihood of success of
treatment is not in fact a morally justifiable selection criterion for
care. There are several reasons for this:

1. We may consider that we should always try to alleviate
symptoms as a point of principle, and that the effort to do so is
valuable in itself. There are two reasons for this. First, it is related to
the ideal that we never say 'There is nothing more I can do', perhaps
because this statement has been seen as indicative of patient
abandonment. It may be that we consider that continuous striving
to alleviate symptoms demonstrates to the patient that we (and
therefore society) still value them, but even if this is true it is hard
to justify denying another patient a scarce resource in order to
demonstrate continuous valuing for one patient. In fact a
compromise is generally reached whereby the patient is likely to be
discharged when all possible has been done towards symptom
control, but the team keep in close contact to monitor needs and
maintain support by their presence. This liberates the resource for
use by others. Secondly, it may be because so much of life seems to
be about the struggle to achieve goals which in the end are rarely
attained, such as the struggle for justice in law, for international
peace, and for fulfilling relationships. We value these ends and so
value the struggle to attain them, possibly because the striving
affirms our commitment to them as well as enabling us to inch
forward slowly towards them.

2. Since the course of the disease and response to treatment in
palliative care is difficult to predict, carers may consider that the
likelihood of success of treatment is so unpredictable as to be
inappropriate as a criterion of selection for specialist care.

3. The benefits of palliative care are without doubt related to the
process of care itself, and not just to therapeutic interventions such
as medication and specific nursing techniques. This benefit is
independent of the success of such interventions. Therefore the likely
success of interventions is too narrow a selection criterion to be used

ve this com-
l relief of
ources
nt

...g *ability to benefit from the process*
...ion, but this would apply to virtually
...for selection at all. Instead we might
... *the process of care*, in the sense of
...if denied that process, as a selection
...ve priority to an isolated paraplegic
...rthlessness related to dependency and
...t from the process of care, even though
...is unlikely to be successful in terms of
re-cost...

We have said that where psychosocial and spiritual care are concerned, it is impossible to differentiate between the benefit derived from the process of care and that derived from specific interventions. Much has been said in the context of palliative care about the value of accompanying patients on their 'emotional and spiritual journeys'. This statement is about commitment to the patient and affirmation of the patient's worth as well as the idea that patients benefit from the process of care.

In summary we might say that in palliative care the criteria of medical utility include patient need and the ability to benefit from both the process of care and the specific interventions of care.

Medical utility is not the only morally justifiable selection criterion. *Opportunity costs* for other patients and *prior commitments* to individual patients are also morally relevant, and the *needs and likelihood of benefit of relatives* may be justifiable criteria in some circumstances.

Opportunity costs arise whenever a patient is using a scarce resource, since that resource is not then available to another patient for whom that resource may have greater medical utility. This becomes relevant in palliative care if transfer of a patient from an acute medical or surgical ward or a specialist cancer centre is requested. The presence of the palliative care patient in such facilities may deny access to other patients who have greater need of their particular resources and who would benefit more from them. Of course the extent of opportunity costs depends on the pressure for beds in the other specialist facilities. It is difficult to give priority to patients in these acute specialist facilities on the grounds that other 'mythical' patients, to whom one does not have an immediate commitment, also require them. Nevertheless, opportunity costs are a morally justifiable selection criterion when there is genuine pressure on the resources of other specialist facilities.

Prior commitments to patients are also morally important, and this is acknowledged by clinical staff who should encourage managerial staff to do likewise. If a patient has been promised access to a facility, be it an in-patient bed, technical procedure, specialist nurse, or social worker time, then that promise should be honoured. Conflicts of conscience then arise if a patient with a greater moral claim on that facility requires it. Moral conflict for professionals is avoided where possible by the simple expedient of avoiding commitments, but this is not entirely satisfactory either. For example, patients may not be told that an in-patient bed is available until the day of admission, in order to be able to prioritize patients for it at the last possible moment, so that maximum benefit can be obtained from its use. This means that patients are kept waiting in anxiety, which would have been lessened considerably if they knew for certain when they could be admitted. Deliberate avoidance of commitment makes rationing easier, but it makes life harder for palliative care patients by burdening their lives with yet more uncertainty. Wherever possible we should make commitments, but then they should be honoured unless an absolutely overwhelming claim of need arises. In other cases of conflict the balance should arguably be given to honouring the commitment.

Social utility is usually defined as the comparative value of the patients who may receive treatment to the community. It is a term used in discussions about selection of patients for life-prolonging or life-sustaining treatments such as renal dialysis and major organ transplants. For example, a young mother of three or a businessman providing major employment might both be given priority over a young drug addict who supports his habit through crime. Whether social utility is or is not just as a selection criterion is simply not relevant in palliative care where life cannot be greatly prolonged or artificially sustained in the long term.

None the less, specialist palliative care does carry benefits for relatives of patients in terms of decreasing physical and emotional burdens. This could be termed the *likelihood of success of care to and for the family* (as distinct from the patient). To what extent should the needs of relatives influence allocation of resources? Whilst our primary commitment is to the welfare of the patient, we do have a secondary commitment to that of relatives. Moreover, the welfare of those around the patient is inextricably mixed with that of the patient. Therefore, if all other patient-related selection criteria are equal, we would allocate the resource to that patient whose relatives are most in need of the benefits of specialist care. Unfortunately, this morally clear case is not the norm in clinical practice, where it is very difficult to judge what priority should be given to patients on the grounds of family need and likelihood of benefit. This moral judgement is always going to be complex and difficult, and in may cases there will be no single 'right' answer. Ultimately, those responsible for selection must make a choice which is morally justifiable, whilst being aware that no choice is ideal, and more than one choice is probably justifiable.

Age has been much discussed as a criterion for discrimination for the purposes of rationing health care. In times of crisis due to shortage of resources age has been used as a selection criterion on the practical basis that it is easy to enforce and on the moral basis that it is easier to meet the needs of older patients outside specialist services, for instance by using highly developed geriatric services. It does not seem reasonable to postulate that the medical needs of the elderly terminally ill are any less than those of younger patients, and indeed they may be greater because of multiple additional pathologies associated with ageing. Emotional and social needs often appear greater in younger patients, but it may also be argued that this is a qualitative rather than a quantitative difference. Once again, it is not possible to weigh different needs in a balance. Younger patients are often given priority over older ones for the simple and morally justifiable reason that the needs of the elderly can often be met through a well-developed geriatric service, whereas there is no comparable service for the young whose needs can therefore be met only by specialist palliative care. It should be noted that this distinction is in fact based on need and not on age.

Queuing, or the law of 'first-come-first-served', is a common system of rationing in health care. However, it does not seem justifiable to regard the accident of timing of referral as a selection criterion for specialist palliative care, unless we are prepared to use luck or chance in the process of selection. In palliative care, where circumstances and needs change rapidly and patients often deteriorate and die quickly, queuing is an unsatisfactory way of rationing services—people simply die on the waiting list without their needs being met. The policy of queuing also means that longevity from the time of referral determines allocation of resources, and this does not seem justifiable. 'Managing' the length of a waiting list by accepting the death of patients on it as a natural selection procedure is not a morally acceptable solution to the problems of rationing specialist palliative care.

Continuous reselection of patients in receipt of specialist care is morally required, and is done on the basis of assessment of need for that specialist service. When resources are scarce, patients whose needs can be met outside the specialist unit are discharged so as to make room for others who will sustain harm if denied access to the specialist service. This does mean that patients who would benefit from remaining in specialist care have to leave it, even if they would rather stay, but this is morally necessary in order to distribute the resource justly.

As the difficult issue of rationing has exercised the minds of palliative care workers for so long, and is now increasingly and rightfully subject to public scrutiny, it has become generally accepted that some selection criteria are not morally justifiable. These include sex, ethnic and cultural background, and religion. It is also considered morally wrong to discriminate against smokers who have lung cancer, or AIDS patients, on the grounds that their lifestyle may have been causally responsible for their illness. In the United Kingdom and many Western countries ability to pay for palliative care is also not considered morally justifiable as a selection criterion.

12.4   Conclusions

1. Health care resources should be allocated and used so as to maximize benefit and distribute that benefit justly.

2. Affluent societies have a strong moral obligation to provide a decent minimum level of palliative care; this entails acquisition of the knowledge and skills required for competence by all health care workers, coupled with morally appropriate attitudes. Some patients require specialist palliative care in order to meet their needs.

3. There is no moral obligation to provide unlimited care, that is every facility which patients might demand or could benefit from. There is a weak obligation to provide more than

adequate care if the society is sufficiently affluent to fund it as a priority, either by enforceable or charitable means.

4. Morally justifiable selection criteria for specialist care are patient need, differential likelihood of benefit or success from interventions and from the process of care, opportunity cost, and prior commitment. Continuous reselection of patients is morally required.

13

Reply to critics

People ask you for criticism, but they only want praise.
Somerset Maugham, *Of Human Bondage*, Ch. 50

It might seem an advantage of a second edition that authors have a chance to consider reviewers' criticisms of their book and improve it in the light of those criticisms. The problem with this approach, however, is that reviewers do not speak with one voice. Indeed, they often contradict each other. Here are a few not unamusing examples. The reviewer in the *University of Toronto Medical Journal* complains of the 'complexity of language and the fact that the authors' perspective was removed and theoretical' and that 'the verbose and rather dry manner in which the information is presented makes it somewhat difficult to read'. On the other hand, the reviewer in *Palliative Medicine* finds that 'the text is readable, concise without being "skimpy"' and the reviewer in *Bioethics* finds the 'writing is clear and the language should be accessible to a wide readership'. The *University of Toronto Medical Journal* thinks that the book 'will probably be reserved for those with a more theoretical interest in the subject, such as medical ethicists', and complains that 'the discussion was from a philosophical and historical viewpoint, which served to complicate the information', whereas his colleague from McGill University writing in *Theoretical Medicine and Bioethics* judges that 'the authors could have made their arguments more convincing had they incorporated more of a philosophical and historical analysis into their conclusions'. The diversity of comments probably reflects the diversity of backgrounds and disciplines from which the reviewers come.

We are of course grateful that the reviewers have taken the trouble to comment on the book, but in view of the contradictory reactions we shall leave the style much as it is, although the addition of more clinical examples should be of interest to those who are less comfortable with unillustrated items.

There are, however, several criticisms we shall take up. This is less because we wish to be defensive about the book than because the reviewers have pointed to areas of important controversy in palliative care. There are three such areas. They are: (1) a more detailed discussion regarding withholding and withdrawing life-prolonging treatment; (2) the moral problems of giving overriding power to the principle of respect for the patient's autonomy; and (3) the provision of spiritual and emotional care.

13.1   The moral distinction between killing and letting die

In Chapter 5, Section 5.3.3, we discussed this distinction briefly, but in view of its importance in palliative care and the continuing public and media interest in the topic we have included in this chapter a further discussion in greater depth. It is important when thinking about this topic that arguments are carried through and their implications for the whole of health care are examined.

In Chapter 5 we concluded that whereas letting die has to be permitted when the burdens and risks of life-prolonging treatment clearly outweigh its benefits, at the same time society needs to maintain its prohibition against killing (murder) in order to protect its members. In order to achieve these two aims the law has to uphold a clear distinction between killing and letting die.

In law an act of killing is murder if one person intended to cause and did cause the death of another. It is prohibited in most cultures, and is severely punished. Thus a charge of murder would be brought against a doctor who intended to cause and did cause the death of a patient. On the other hand, a doctor who withholds or withdraws a life-prolonging treatment from a patient because its burdens and risks outweigh its benefits, or because the patient refuses the treatment, is considered to have allowed a foreseen death to occur from natural causes and is not charged with murder. In this situation letting the patient die is legally permitted. Unfortunately, the advent of technology has made the moral distinction between killing and letting die appear very blurred in some cases. There are two reasons for this.

The first reason is to do with ambiguity around the cause of death. It is sometimes argued that the withdrawal of life-prolonging or life-sustaining treatment *causes* the death of the patient, and causing the death of the patient is one of the two conditions for murder. For example, when life-prolonging treatments such as artificial feeding and hydration are removed from patients in the persistent vegetative state (PVS), or artificial ventilation is removed from stable but unconscious ventilator-dependent patients, it is overwhelmingly likely that death will follow, and so some people consider that such withdrawal of life-prolonging treatment actually causes the patient's death. They therefore think that it should be considered morally and legally to be the cause of the patient's death.

On the other hand, we would wish to argue that the patient's death is caused by the underlying failure of essential organ function (for example, permanent unconsciousness or inability to breathe) which renders the patient incapable of survival without constant life-prolonging treatment. The fundamental cause of death is the patient's condition, not the withdrawal of treatment, which should be regarded as incidental. Death would have been caused by the pathological conditions of the PVS or inability to breathe. The life-support treatments merely prevent on a temporary basis the occurrence of death. Such temporary measures give doctors time to assess the situation and to consider whether the body can resume normal functioning or whether there is reasonable hope of improvement. If in these situations there is no reasonable hope of recovery of consciousness or the ability to breath, further life-sustaining treatment cannot confer benefit and therefore it is not in the patient's interests to continue it. When it is removed the body's own causality results in death.

If our line of reasoning is rejected and it is considered instead that doctors cause the death of patients when they switch off ventilators or remove artificial nutrition and hydration from patients in the PVS, then it must follow that in all cases where doctors have withdrawn life-prolonging treatment for any reason they have caused the patient's death. Since the available array of life-prolonging treatment is so extensive, and since the precise timing of so many patients' deaths is now influenced by decisions to forgo some possible life-prolonging technology, one would have to conclude that doctors actually cause the death of the majority of their terminally ill patients. For example, one would have to conclude that doctors cause the patient's death whenever they discontinue a cardiopulmonary resuscitation attempt because technically the doctors could have supported the patient's circulation artificially for some time longer. Such a conclusion is deeply counter-intuitive.

Furthermore, if one considers as we do that there is no necessary moral difference between withholding and withdrawing a life-prolonging treatment, one would have to conclude that when doctors withhold a life-prolonging treatment in a terminal illness, such as artificial ventilation in motor neurone disease, or renal dialysis and artificial nutrition and hydration in those terminally ill, they are causing the death of those patients, because they have withheld a treatment which for a limited time could technically have prolonged life. Similarly, the withholding of antibiotics for pneumonia for patients with a very poor prognosis would also be regarded as tantamount to causing the patients death (if it is thought antibiotics might have prolonged life). Such a conclusion is also deeply counter-intuitive.

Moreover, if doctors were considered to have caused the patient's death whenever they withheld or withdrew life-prolonging treatment, the law would have to examine each incident as a possible case of murder. If it were judged that the doctor might have intended the death of the patient (which he or she was considered to have caused), then a charge of murder would have to be made. This situation would be completely unmanageable legally. But if withholding and withdrawing life-prolonging treatment is considered to cause death, this unmanageable legal situation could be avoided only if the prohibition against intentionally causing death were abolished. Such an alteration in the law would be highly undesirable because it would remove an essential protection for all members of society.

The second reason for the blurring of the moral distinction between killing and letting die is to do with the distinction between intending and foreseeing the outcome of a decision. The moral distinction between intending and foreseeing the death of the patient following withholding or withdrawal of life-prolonging treatment may be finely drawn. For example, it is sometimes argued that when a doctor switches off a ventilator-dependent patient's ventilator, or removes artificial feeding and hydration from a patient in the PVS, that doctor is intending to cause the patient's death. Those who take this position assert that the doctor must inevitably intend the patient's death since he or she knows that it is overwhelmingly likely that death will follow withdrawal of these treatments. The contrary position, which we would hold, is that the doctor intends only to withdraw a futile and non-beneficial treatment, and foresees but does not intend the patient's death.

There are two aspects to intention in this case. The first is to do with what the doctor wants, desires, or seeks as the outcome of the decision. Some people who maintain that the doctor intends the patient's death seem to believe that the doctor wants or desires the patient's death. Yet this is surely not the most accurate representation of the case. The doctor is in no way seeking the patient's death, even if it is agreed that death is the least bad outcome because it is considered preferable to continued existence in a state of profound disability, distress, or discomfort. The representation which we feel most accurately describes the case is that the doctor neither desires nor seeks the patients death, but rather intends only to withdraw or withhold a non-beneficial and possibly burdensome treatment. No doctor should seek a patient's death, but equally no doctor wants (or should want) to impose a treatment which confers no benefit and which may be burdensome.

The second aspect of intention relates to the fact that it is intention *to cause* the death of the patient which is being considered. Thus those who believe that the doctor who withdraws or withholds life-prolonging treatment intends the patient's death must believe that the doctor intends *to cause* the patient's death. We contend that since doctors quite reasonably do not consider that the withdrawal or withholding of life-prolonging treatment is the fundamental cause of the patient's death, they cannot logically intend to cause death by withholding or withdrawing treatment. It makes no sense to say that doctors intend to cause death when they do not think their decision is the cause of that death.

In summary, then, we consider that doctors who withhold or withdraw life-prolonging treatment when its burdens outweigh its benefits neither cause nor intend to cause the patient's death. It seems to us that the most accurate representation of the moral situation is to say that they withhold or withdraw treatment which they consider is inappropriate because its burdens exceed its benefits, and that they foresee the patient's death but do not desire or seek it, or intend to cause it.

We have now examined the source of the difficulties in the distinction between killing and letting die in the medical context. We have argued for our view on the grounds that there are counter-intuitive aspects and bad consequences of the view that doctors intentionally cause the deaths of patients when they withhold or withdraw life-prolonging treatment. However, since this is one of the many moral questions on which opinions differ, some people will inevitably disagree with us, and those who do sometimes develop an argument to suggest that the legal prohibition of 'mercy killing' should be revoked. (In this context we define mercy killing or euthanasia as an intentional act which causes the death of the patient and which is done through compassionate motives.) They argue that there is no significant moral difference between intentionally causing the death of a patient (mercy killing or euthanasia) and withholding or withdrawing life-prolonging treatment (acts fitting our description of letting die). In other words they assert that letting die is morally indistinguishable from euthanasia or mercy killing. They also assert that the law should treat acts which are considered morally indistinguishable in the same way, so that if letting die is permitted so should acts of mercy killing or euthanasia be permitted. Their arguments can be presented as a logical syllogism as follows:

Major premise: Morally indistinguishable cases should not be treated differently by law.

Minor premise: Acts of letting die are morally indistinguishable from acts of mercy killing or euthanasia.

Conclusion: Therefore the law should not treat acts of mercy killing or euthanasia differently from acts of letting die.

Whilst the conclusion does follow logically from the premises, we would contend that the premises are seriously flawed and so the conclusion based on them should be rejected.

The minor premise has already been examined above, where we concluded that there are important moral differences between acts of letting die and acts of mercy killing or euthanasia. Therefore they are not morally indistinguishable and so the minor premise is false. We concluded above that the moral differences lie both in intention and in causation of death; in cases of 'letting die' the doctors neither intend to cause nor cause the death of the patient whereas in acts of mercy killing they both intend to cause and do cause the death of the patient.

The major premise, that morally indistinguishable cases should not be treated differently by law, raises issues about the function of law and its relationship to morality. Three essential points should be considered. First, it should be remembered that the function of the law is to safeguard the interests of everyone in the community and not just the interests of a minority, however deserving, against the majority. Secondly, morality is much more complex than the law could ever be. An enforceable, consistent, and comprehensible law is necessarily a relatively 'blunt instrument' compared with the great complexity of moral judgements. Yet it is with this blunt instrument that the good of the community must be upheld. So the law has to make distinctions which are unambiguous and comprehensible to ordinary folk, and it cannot possibly follow all the intricacies and nuances of thought and feeling which exist in morality. Thirdly, in treating acts of letting die differently from mercy killing or euthanasia the law is not saying that there is *always* a moral difference between letting die and killing. It is saying only that for legal purposes related to the best outcome for the whole community it is necessary to make this distinction. Indeed, the purpose of law is not to say which acts are or are not morally indistinguishable. In addition, we would argue that in general there is a significant moral difference between acts of mercy killing and letting die, although it may be possible to produce scenarios where there is no significant moral difference. It follows from all of these considerations that it is likely that there will be unusual occasions when morally indistinguishable cases will have to be treated differently by law, in the interests of everyone in the community. Although at first sight this situation appears morally undesirable, it is not wrong if the good of everyone requires it. Moreover, it appears to us that whether it is right or wrong, this situation is probably unavoidable.

We have asserted that both premises are false. Nevertheless, if they are accepted by some people the conclusion will logically follow, and so we should consider the consequences of accepting the conclusion. The conclusion suggests that letting die and mercy killing or euthanasia should not be treated differently in law. This would mean treating intentional acts of 'causing death' in the same way as acts of withholding or withdrawing life-prolonging treatment in the context of allowing to die. It would follow then that either both should be prohibited, or both should be permitted.

We have already argued that disastrous consequences for patients would ensue if the withholding or withdrawing of life-prolonging treatment were prohibited. All patients would then be allowed to die only after the application of all possible means to prolong life. Indeed, the phrase 'allowed to die' would no longer have any application; patients would in fact die if and only if they defeated the medical technology! This would have disastrous results; the autonomy of patients and doctors would be grossly infringed by the law, life-prolonging treatments could not be withheld or withdrawn even if their harms outweighed their benefits, thus increasing suffering, and intensive care units would consume the lion's share of the community's resources for health care.

In fact it is much more common to hear it argued that both letting die and mercy killing should be permitted. For example, it might be suggested that withdrawal of feeding from patients in the PVS is morally indistinguishable from euthanasia and that both should be permitted. The consequences of such a view must be examined. Proponents of this view would contend that when doctors withdraw feeding from a PVS patient they have intentionally caused the death of the patient because they consider that the patient's quality of life is so poor that he or she should not be kept alive. They would then conclude that if allowing to die is permitted for this reason in the PVS cases, then voluntary and indeed non-voluntary euthanasia for the same reason must also be permitted. This would mean that if it was thought that a person's quality of life was considered so poor that he or she should not be kept alive by means of life-prolonging treatment, then a deliberate act to cause the death of that person should also be permitted. It would then follow that doctors, and indeed perhaps anyone, would be permitted to kill such patients. This would severely weaken the prohibition against killing which currently protects such vulnerable patients.

Sometimes the argument for permitting both letting die and killing is carried further, and it is then suggested that there is a moral obligation to administer lethal injections to patients whose quality of life doctors feel is so poor that life-prolonging interventions should be withheld or withdrawn. We will explore the consequences of such a view because it is quite often put forward in discussions on this subject. If this view is to be upheld by law, it follows that the law should consider that there may be a moral obligation to give lethal injections to such patients because it is considered more humane that omitting life-prolonging treatment such as feeding. The argument can be presented in the following logical syllogism:

Major premise: There is a moral obligation in medical practice to act only in the most humane way.

Minor premise: It is more humane to give patients with a poor quality of life a lethal injection than to withdraw life-prolonging treatment.

Conclusion: There is a moral obligation to give patients with a poor quality of life a lethal injection.

Once again, the conclusion does follow logically from the premises, but the premises themselves are flawed.

The major premise is oversimplistic. The moral life in medical practice is more complex than this. When making laws, society must have regard to the requirement for the most humane treatment for *all* patients. When making decisions regarding the treatment of an individual patient, doctors must have regard to the rules established to promote humane treatment for all. We would argue that in the interests of providing the most humane treatment possible, bearing in mind the circumstances of *all* patients, the prohibition against giving lethal injections to patients deemed to have a poor quality of life must be maintained.

The minor premise is also open to dispute. For example, it is dangerously misleading to make emotive statements about the suffering of patients in the PVS. It is sometimes suggested that such patients 'starve to death' if feeding is withdrawn. But the term 'starve to death' is a phrase associated with a painful state of consciousness which is not thought to be present in such patients. It is generally considered that patients in the PVS do not perceive hunger or thirst. Moreover, in other instances where life-prolonging treatment is withheld or withdrawn in other clinical conditions, for instance regarding ventilation, the patient may continue to breathe and thus not die. This may turn out to be a more humane outcome than having life ended by a lethal injection.

The conclusion of this syllogism, that there is a moral obligation to give patients who have a poor quality of life a lethal injection, will be unpalatable to most readers.

We have analysed the arguments above in detail to illustrate that it is essential that arguments about the moral and legal distinctions between acts of killing and letting die must be conducted thoroughly and logically, and the consequences of the conclusions must be followed through in terms of the good of the whole of society. Many books have been written on the subject of euthanasia, and currently debate continues about whether it should be permitted in law. In this context our argument is simply to the effect that there is no logical connection between withholding and withdrawing treatment, intending and foreseeing the patient's death on the one hand, and euthanasia on the other.

13.2   The problems of supremacy of patient autonomy

Some critics of the first edition of this book have suggested that our approach resulted in what they consider to be unjustifiable infringement of the patient's autonomy. Presumably this criticism arose because we advocated that health care professionals should refuse to provide treatments requested by patients if the professionals considered that in the circumstances those treatments would confer overall harm, or if to provide them would deprive other patients of more beneficial treatment. At the root of this criticism lies a very important debate about the appropriate scope and authority of the principle of respect for the patient's autonomy in health care ethics. Therefore in this chapter we shall discuss in some depth the question of whether the principle of respect for the patient's autonomy should have overriding power when conflicts arise between it and the other principles.

In Chapter 1 we stated that no single principle has overriding authority in relation to the others. The principles represent duties of equal importance; when conflict arises between them, the individual must weigh up the morally relevant factors and then decide which principle should override in those particular circumstances. In addition, we have described clinical situations where we believe that there are certain limitations to the application of each principle. For example, the principle of respect for the patient's autonomy cannot require the doctor to provide a treatment which the doctor strongly believes will not further the patient's medical good or which will actually cause overall harm. On the other hand, the principle of beneficence does not entitle doctors to force a treatment on a competent patient who is refusing it. Since no principle has overriding power and there are limitations to their application, a balance is struck between principles in the clinical situation. We believe that it is essential for the promotion of the good of present and future patients that this balance be preserved in the 'philosophy of palliative care'. Unfortunately, current trends in health care ethics and the general rise of consumerism and individualism in society are putting this delicate balance at risk.

From the beginning of the development of palliative care there has been explicit acknowledgement that the autonomy of the patient should be respected in terms of knowledge of the diagnosis and prognosis, and choice in terms of appropriate treatment and the place and mode of dying where possible. At the same time, health care professionals have upheld the importance of the principles of beneficence and non-maleficence. This is illustrated by their refusal to provide futile but requested treatment to patients. It is also generally agreed that a treatment ought not to be provided for one patient if to do so would deprive another patient of a more effective and needed treatment. Thus a balance between the principles of justice, beneficence, non-maleficence, and respect for autonomy has been maintained until the mid-1990s.

However, recently, a new movement has been born in health care and we could call this the 'supremacy of patient autonomy' move-ment. It is closely linked to the increasing tendency to regard patients and their relatives as consumers of health care in a market economy model. Unfortunately, the original philosophy of palliative care is perhaps being overtaken, hijacked, or swamped by the enthusiasm for this new 'supremacy of patient autonomy' movement, to the extent that it may even be thought that the aim of health care is the promotion of patients' autonomy (as opposed to their health). This movement has very serious consequences for patients and health care professionals today and in the future.

There are several reasons for the current tendency to regard respect for the patient's autonomy as the overriding principle and we have discussed these in Chapter 1.

The social background against which this development in health care ethics has occurred is not likely to change quickly. In other words, enthusiasm for what is new, along with consumerism and individualism, is likely to remain for a time, and people will always seek some way of resolving moral conflict easily by establishing a single overriding principle. Thus the causes of the rise of the 'supremacy of patient autonomy' movement will remain, so that it is likely to take over health care ethics unless compelling reasons are evident to cause the public and health care professionals to resist it. We shall consider first whether such reasons exist, secondly whether they are generally appreciated, and lastly whether they are sufficiently compelling to require us to resist and oppose the 'supremacy of patient autonomy' movement in health care and palliative care ethics.

13.2.1   *Why should we oppose the establishment of respect for the patient's autonomy as the overriding principle in health care?*

The simplest approach is to consider whether there might be adverse consequences to patients of giving this principle overriding power such that the doctor's overriding duty is always to do what the patient wants. The following adverse consequences are foreseeable and already evident to a certain extent in clinical practice.

The first problem is that this principle is absolutely no help when making decisions about treatment and care for non-autonomous patients, such as those who are confused, demented, or unconscious. In the context of palliative care, patients are very often non-autonomous for a period, especially at the very end of life. When the patient is non-autonomous, the consequence of giving this principle overriding power is that professionals seek the autonomy of some other person to respect. They therefore tend to make respecting the autonomy of the relatives their guiding principle, rather than acting in the patient's best interest. There are two obvious problems with this: the relatives' expressed wishes may not reflect the wishes the patient would have expressed in the circumstances, and doing what the relatives want may not advance the patient's medical good. This means that just when the dying and uncommunicative patient needs us as an advocate (to use popular jargon) we in fact do what the relatives want rather than what is in the patient's best interest if a clash between the two occurs. It is ironic that a direct result of making the principle of respect for the patient's autonomy the overriding principle is that non-autonomous patients may suffer harm.

The likelihood of this result is increased by the fact that it is human nature to try to avoid difficult conflict. It is undoubtedly easier to comply with the relatives' wishes than to uphold the patient's best interests and thus have to spend considerable time and effort explaining and justifying our decisions to the relatives, a process which many doctors find stressful and perhaps threatening.

In a sense, making respect for the patient's autonomy an overriding principle almost encourages professionals to take the 'easy way out' and comply with the wishes of the relatives' of non-autonomous patients even when doing so does not accord with the patient's best interests. Courage is often required when upholding the interests of non-autonomous patients.

A second and related adverse consequence is that the wishes and needs of autonomous patients tend to be given precedence over the needs of non-autonomous patients whose wishes are not known. This is a logical consequence of giving the principle of respect for the wishes of autonomous patients overriding power, because the principles of beneficence, non-maleficence, and justice must be seen as of lesser importance. Yet these principles are essential in ensuring that the best interests of non-autonomous patients are upheld. If they are considered less important, then logically preference must be given to respecting the wishes of autonomous patients as opposed to upholding the best interests of non-autonomous patients. It is also a natural consequence of human nature that the needs of autonomous patients are given preference over those of non-autonomous patients, especially when resources are constrained, for non-autonomous patients are not able to complain about injustices. Professionals naturally want to avoid having to deal with complaints from patients, and only autonomous patients are in a position to complain.

A third adverse consequence of health care professionals considering that their overriding duty is to do what patients want is that patients may be harmed. For example, patients are likely to sustain overall harm when doctors provide treatment such as non-curative chemotherapy even when they know that its overall harms and risks exceed the possible benefits, but they give it because the patient requests any treatment which carries a chance of prolonging life. Judgements about treatment in health care must always be made in the light of the particular clinical circumstances, and treatments which would be beneficial in some clinical situations are actually harmful or excessively risky in others. But if the principle of respect for the patient's autonomy is given overriding power in relation to those of beneficence and non-maleficence, then professionals must provide whatever treatment the patient requests. Thus in those unusual cases where patients request a treatment, even when informed that professionals consider its harms and risks outweigh its benefits, they would then receive the treatment, leading to overall harm.

A fourth problem follows indirectly from the third and it relates to the concepts of harm and benefit themselves. When the principle of respect for the patient's autonomy is given overriding power, professionals tend to think that doing what the patient wants is necessarily a benefit to the patient, and conversely that not doing what the patient requests is necessarily a harm to the patient. In other words, 'harm' and 'benefit' are seen to be totally subjective concepts with no important objective content. We allude to this problem in Chapter 14 on quality of life. If decisions are ever to be made for non-autonomous patients (who have not made an advance statement), there must be some objective content to the concepts of harm and benefit.

A fifth adverse consequence, therefore, is that respect for the patient's autonomy comes to be seen as the goal of health care. One reason for rejecting this conclusion outright, especially in the context of palliative care, is that it leads one to believe that there is no possible health care goal for patients who are not autonomous and have no future prospect of regaining their autonomy!

The sixth adverse consequence is that health care professionals lose their sense of moral responsibility for the outcome of the treatment they provide. This is an understandable and logical consequence because, to a great extent, decision-making responsibility has effectively been passed to the patient. Until the present time, doctors have considered that they should offer to patients only those treatments which they consider may offer overall benefit, and they have not offered treatments which they consider offer no benefit or which are associated with harms and risks which are excessive in comparison with the benefit in the particular clinical circumstances. Doctors have also frequently offered advice about which of the offered treatments would be best in the patient's case. However, if respect for the patient's autonomy is to be the overriding principle, doctors will tend to think they should offer *all possible* treatments, and then provide whichever treatment the patient chooses. This may sound implausible, but there is evidence that doctors are already beginning to believe that this policy is right. For example, some consider that they should discuss cardiopulmonary resuscitation with all patients and provide it for all who then request it, even for those patients for whom the evidence shows that there is virtually no chance of success and that it is virtually certain that a resuscitation attempt will result only in an undignified and traumatic death. This scenario illustrates the emergence of a situation in which decision-making authority has passed completely to the patient, and so health care professionals quite reasonably lose any sense of moral responsibility for the outcome of the treatment provided. Health care will have become a service industry, as we suggested in Chapter 1.

The eighth consequence of giving respect for the patient's autonomy overriding power is that legalization of voluntary euthanasia would tend to follow as a logical development (unless other social reasons for prohibiting it were considered compelling). If the principle of respect for the patient's autonomy were considered to override those of beneficence and non-maleficence, it would become a doctor's duty to end patients' lives at their request, as is very frequently argued at present. This would apply even if the patients were not physically ill, but were mentally wretched for some reason and wanted life ended. Those who are opposed to the practice and legalization of euthanasia would consider this to be an adverse consequence to society.

The ninth problem arises in the context of publicly funded health care services where rationing is essential. If the principle of respect for the patient's autonomy is seen to have overriding power in relation to that of justice, it follows that patients who request a treatment must receive it even if the result is unjust deprivation of other patients, such as non-autonomous patients. In fact this adverse consequence is usually obvious to the public and to health care professionals, and so there seems to be general agreement that where health care is publicly funded, there will be occasions when a patient cannot receive a requested treatment because of shortage of resources, including non-financial resources such as donated organs.

The tenth adverse consequence is perhaps morally the most serious for society, for it is the tendency to locate the value or worth of human beings in their autonomy. If the overriding principle of health care is considered to be the promotion of and respect for the autonomy of patients, then people tend to think that being autonomous is what makes a human being valuable, or gives him or her 'worth'. Unfortunately, the corollary of this is that human beings who are and will remain substantially less autonomous than others, or those who have become non-autonomous in the process of dying, are seen as less valuable. It is then only one small step to making them expendable in the interests of the autonomous (see Chapter 3).

It may be argued that these ten adverse consequences paint an unreasonably black picture which might never actually occur. However, we have argued that the process of logic combined with human nature will tend to lead to all of them, and we consider that together they constitute a major harm to society and especially to the sick.

A similarly daunting list of adverse consequences could be drawn up in relation to giving any of the other principles overriding power, although one could argue at length about which list would constitute the least of evils! The point is that where these principles are used as a way of considering moral problems in palliative care, they must be considered to have equal intrinsic importance or power.

So far our reasons for opposing the 'supremacy of patient autonomy' movement have been based on the adverse consequences of such a policy. However, there is also an important philosophical argument against establishing a principle of respect for *the patient's* autonomy as an overriding principle. This argument rests on the philosophical basis of the principle of respect for autonomy, namely that the principle is *universally* applicable. In other words, respect for their autonomy is deserved by all autonomous people equally. Thus respect for the patient's autonomy must coexist with respect for the autonomy of health care professionals and others in the patient's circle. Respect for the autonomy of health care professionals requires that they cannot be forced by a principle of respect for autonomy to do things to patients which they believe will confer overall harm on those patients.

Furthermore, it can be argued that health care professionals who are inevitably entrusted with the welfare of vulnerable people should not be expected or even allowed to act in ways which they believe are harmful to those people. This reflects the concept of the caring role of health professionals, which requires them to have and to continue to develop a natural tendency to benefit patients and to protect them from harm. It is hardly possible to develop and maintain this tendency if at the same time those professionals are required to give treatments, even at the request of patients, which they consider to be harmful in the circumstances. This point affirms our previous argument that the principle of respect for autonomy applies to all autonomous people, and so is universal—it does not apply only to patients.

13.2.2 Are the above reasons generally appreciated?

It is difficult to say whether the adverse consequences of the 'supremacy of patient autonomy' idea are generally appreciated. Certainly the difficulty of emphasizing the importance of respect for patient autonomy, whilst at the same time opposing the legalization of voluntary euthanasia, is recognized. In addition, most people seem to accept that where resources are limited, the requirements of justice sometimes dictate that individual patient requests must be overridden. On the other hand, there seems to be little discussion of the problems which arise when the concepts of harm and benefit lose objective content, and professionals and the public come to consider that whatever the patient wants is necessarily beneficial. Currently, any allusion to the autonomy of the professional, or to the duties to benefit patients in a medical sense and avoid medical harm to them, is unpopular. It is thought inevitably to indicate willingness to infringe the patient's autonomy. Any such infringement tends to be considered as necessarily unjustifiable. Hence the term 'paternalistic' has come to have derogatory overtones which are in stark contrast to the image of loving fatherly actions.

It is not surprising that the fact that the principle of respect for autonomy is universalizable seems not to be generally appreciated by health care professionals. The latter will probably have heard of the principle only in relation to the patient's autonomy in the context of health care ethics, and they are likely to be unaware of its philosophical roots and its application to all autonomous persons. They are much more likely to be under the (mistaken) impression that patients have some kind of indefeasible right, that is a right which cannot be overruled, to any treatment which they might request.

13.2.3 Are the reasons sufficiently compelling to require us to oppose the establishment of the principle of respect for the patient's autonomy as an overriding principle?

It is our view that since the duty to respect the autonomy of the patient was first promoted in palliative care, the emphasis on it has become excessive in relation to other health care duties such as benefiting and not harming patients and allocating resources justly. We believe that such undue emphasis will lead to the above adverse consequences which should now be recognized and discussed in the context of health care in general. It is certainly imperative that they are discussed in the context of palliative care where most patients pass through periods when they are non-autonomous and very vulnerable, where the end of life is near and there is little or no opportunity to correct decisions which have led to a bad outcome for the patient, and where the wishes of the relatives are considered to be of such great importance that they may easily override the good of the patient.

We therefore conclude on the basis of the adverse consequences and the universal application of the principle of respect for autonomy that there are compelling reasons why we should oppose the current popular idea that the principle of respect for the patient's autonomy should have intrinsic authority to override the other principles in health care. Our view is that it is imperative that we reflect on the meaning and the appropriate place of the principle of respect for autonomy in health care and particularly in palliative care.

13.3 Emotional care

The majority of reviewers commented on our reservations about emotional, spiritual, and psychological care. One thought we were unnecessarily 'picking a fight' but the majority thought it was good to have such matters aired, even if it did raise a few hackles. In a sense we *were* picking a fight, because in palliative care there can be a bland assumption that emotional care is obviously a good thing. We are really challenging this assumption for two reasons.

The less radical reason is our insistence that from the ethical point of view, emotional care requires its own consent from the patient like any other offered health care. It is quite wrong to tie symptom control to emotional care, so that patients are led to think that they must put up with intrusive questioning about their relationships and fears in order to have their pain managed. Obviously, if a patient is clinically depressed, as distinct from appropriately sad, then this is a symptom which can and should be treated. Equally obviously, if a patient asks to see a chaplain or other spiritual adviser then this must be arranged. But not all patients need or desire such interventions; perhaps they should be left in peace.

More radically, we question whether there is anything which can be called an 'expertise' in emotional care. Courses in 'counselling' now abound and are applied to every area of life. Some types of counselling—such as genetic counselling—have a knowledge base, but non-directive free-floating counselling does not seem to be very effective (Wesley 1996). Indeed, it can be argued that in so far as it creates the impression that ordinary people cannot cope with their own or their relatives' and friends' life-crises, it is patronizing and demoralizing. Patients sometimes have stories to tell which are helpful for diagnosis and treatment, and listening to them may also assist in establishing a relationship of trust with the patient. Indeed, it may be therapeutic or at least comforting for patients to tell their stories (Macnaughton 1996a). But long sessions exploring emotions may make matters worse rather than better, and in wasting words may waste valuable clinical time (Brewin 1998), or indeed the even more valuable time of a life coming to an end.

14

Quality and value of life

The value of life lies not in the length of days but in the use you make of them.

Montaigne, *Essais*, Bk 1, Ch. 20

Discussions of the value of life, or of what makes human life worthwhile, tend to be confined to philosophical contexts. Nevertheless, presuppositions about what that value consists of underlie the withholding or withdrawal of many medical treatments. On the other hand, discussions about quality of life tend to take place in a medical context and can easily become distorted because of the deep-rooted desire of medical researchers to quantify what is inherently qualitative. Moreover, discussions of quality of life are rarely linked with those of the value of life, but clearly there must be a link. Indeed, it is arguable that the value of a life consists just in this, that that life has a certain number of distinctively human qualities. In this concluding chapter we shall attempt an analysis of the two concepts of 'value of life' and 'quality of life', the connections between them, and their bearing on our main theme of the ethics of palliative care. It will emerge that these concepts have directed the approaches we have taken to many issues, such as treatment decisions and rationing. Let us begin with an initial examination of the idea of a value.

14.1 Values and valuing

If we ask 'What is the value of that house, or that painting?' it is clear what we are asking, because the whole context of the question is clear. But this kind of analogy does not usually help with the question 'What is the value of a life?', although sometimes it may, as when a ransom is offered for a captured king.

Some thinkers, who sense the problematic nature of the question, answer it by saying either that life has an infinite value, or that it has an intrinsic value, or that it is valuable 'for its own sake'. The idea of infinite value is not very clear outside mathematics, and it may indeed be dangerously misleading if it is taken to suggest that there is no limit to the resources which may justifiably be expended in keeping someone alive. It is possible, however, to give a meaning to 'intrinsic value' or valuable 'for its own sake'. These expressions can be explained if we draw a contrast between means and ends. Some things or activities are valuable as a means to something else, for example practising scales is a means to becoming a good musician. But other things or activities are valuable as ends, or for their own sakes, or intrinsically, for example being able to play a musical instrument. So we could say that while a job might be a means to a good life, life itself is valuable as an end, or intrinsically, or for its own sake, and not as a means to something else. Now this is clear as far as it goes, but it does not go far enough, for it does not tell us what it is about life which makes it valuable for its own sake.

The temptation here is to say that we cannot progress unless we know what values are. Certainly, questions of the form 'What is X?' are familiar to anyone who has taken a philosophy course. This form of question was introduced by Plato whose Dialogues are concerned with questions such as 'What is knowledge?', 'What is love?', 'What is courage?', 'What is justice?', and so on. The hope is to find a definition, in the form of a set of necessary and sufficient conditions, which will demarcate and distinguish the given concept from related ones. What emerges from such discussions is that the concepts cannot be fully understood without placing them in a total view of the nature of human life. And the same is true of a fundamental concept like 'value'.

Sometimes, however, the way ahead is not to persevere with a difficult question, but to change the question. The philosopher Wittgenstein (1953) describes a fly in a bottle. It constantly buzzes against the glass and cannot escape. But there is no stopper on the bottle; all the fly needs to do is to change direction and it will escape. Let us therefore try changing the direction of the question. Instead of asking 'What is a value?' we shall ask 'What is it to value something?' We have moved from the noun to the verb, to the activity of valuing.

To value something is to choose it (in some way) in preference to something else. Valuing is basically a comparative activity. If we go down this route we can now ask 'What activities or qualities do people tend to choose out of preference to have in their lives?' The answer will give some hints of what it is about life which makes life valuable to people. It is clear that there will be no one quality or activity which everyone will choose, but health, friends, love, and interesting things to do would be typical on any list. Of course, if there were one thing all these items had in common then we might have a short answer to what makes life valuable. A favourite among philosophers from the earliest has been 'rationality', since rationality is that capacity without which the others cannot be exercised. More recently, philosophers, and now the vast majority of doctors and health care ethicists, prefer the term 'autonomy' for expressing what is both distinctive of and uniquely valuable in human beings. 'Autonomy' is preferred to 'rationality' on the grounds that it encapsulates both rationality and the capacity to follow up preferences. (At least this is how 'autonomy' has come to be used, although it is certainly not how Kant, who first made the concept central to personality, interpreted it.) The problem here is that to make 'autonomy' central to what is valuable in human beings leaves the non-autonomous human being in an unclear position. This is especially a problem in palliative care, or in some sorts of psychiatric care, where autonomy may be partly or wholly lacking in some patients. Are they then to be regarded as totally without value?

Some philosophers have suggested that 'consciousness' is what is both distinctive and valuable in human beings. But consciousness seems more like a means than an end; we must be conscious of something, and it is the 'something' which gives the value to consciousness. So we are stuck with a typical list of qualities, capacities, and activities which people tend to choose as giving value to their lives.

We now have the link between the value of life and the quality of life. A life has value to the extent that it possesses at least some of the qualities which people tend to choose out of preference to have in their lives, or which they typically preserve and develop. Some important questions arise here. For example, if a life lacks such typically chosen qualities does that mean it is worthless, and if so, what should then be done about it? Before discussing such controversial questions we shall examine in more detail the idea of 'quality of life'.

14.2 Quality of life

Whereas discussions of the value of life are conducted in the decent obscurity of philosophy books, those on quality of life can be found in medical and nursing texts and journals. Indeed there is a large literature on the concept, including many attempts to develop a quality of life 'scale'. Let us first note briefly some of the contexts in which the concept is used in medicine.

A typical context would be one concerned with the withholding or withdrawing of treatment. For example, consider the following typical case. 'This patient of mine aged 75 is in the terminal stages of Alzheimer's disease. Her quality of life is nil, and she has been like this for five years. Her husband is aware of the situation and his health is declining through cardiac causes and stress. Recently this lady developed an upper respiratory infection and was febrile. Is it ethically acceptable to withhold medication in this case?' In this case the doctor clearly thinks that the ethics of the decision to withhold treatment turn on the question of the quality of life of the patient.

Another range of cases in which quality of life estimates might be involved would be those where a doctor has to arbitrate between the competing claims of patients for scarce resources. For example, there may be competition for a kidney or a liver transplant, and the potential quality of life of the patients involved may be invoked as a basis for the decision. Again, sometimes the wishes of the patient may be in conflict with medical opinion. For example, a doctor may (correctly) judge that the patient's medical condition requires further hospital treatment, but the patient may claim that her quality of life will be better if she returns home. Yet another context in which quality of life judgments are made is the selective non-treatment of neonates. It might be argued that the quality of life of some brain-damaged neonates will be so poor that they should not be treated for treatable conditions.

The idea of 'quality of life' is used so frequently in medical contexts, and has occasioned so much theoretical literature in medical journals, that it is easy to overlook the important point that the term is also used in more general contexts. For example, there is sometimes discussion of the extent to which quality of life in cities is marred by pollution or too many cars. Or there may be debate over whether the quality of life of a society requires the existence of wildernesses, or subsidized arts, or improved architecture.

It should be clear from these problems in medical and wider social decision making that questions of the quality of life overlap with those of happiness, well-being, welfare, and even of what constitutes a meaningful life. But what exactly is the relationship among these concepts? Are they all synonymous? For example, are the components of a meaningful life the same as those of one of good quality? Or are some components subsets of others? For example, are well-being and welfare parts of a life of good quality? Or are some of the concepts rivals? Is a happy life a rival idea to one of good quality? For example, some great historical figures, such as Van Gogh and Beethoven, had lives of good quality, but perhaps not happy lives. These questions call for an answer if we are to have any sort of systematic understanding of 'quality of life' and its bearing on 'value of life'.

Finally, there is the question of who decides on what counts as a life of good quality. Can questions of quality of life be decided by expert or authoritative figures, such as doctors, architects, environmentalists, or politicians? Or is it a matter for democratic, majority voting? Or is it just up to individuals? For example, is it all right for a patient to say, 'I just know that this treatment will improve my quality of life, and I want to have it no matter what the cost'? Again, is it just a matter for majority voting whether or how far there should be public subsidy of the arts?

Questions of this sort can easily induce a sense of despair about the possibility of ever achieving agreed criteria for basing decisions on quality of life judgements. As we shall see, this despair is justifiable. The reasons for it, however, are instructive and in order to identify them we shall employ a method common in philosophy but less accepted in practical spheres such as medicine—that of employing an imaginary situation and developing it. We shall examine and develop the Greek myth of Sisyphus.

14.3 Sisyphus

In Greek mythology Sisyphus was King of Corinth and was known as 'the wily', which is why some stories describe him as the father of Odysseus. For reasons not entirely clear, Sisyphus fell into disfavour with Zeus. One version of the story is that Zeus abducted Aegina, daughter of the river god Asopus. Sisyphus knew the whereabouts of Aegina and disclosed them to Asopus on condition that Asopus would set a river running through Corinth. Zeus was enraged and sent the god of death, Morpheus, to Sisyphus. Sisyphus, however, succeeded in binding Morpheus in chains, and nobody was able to die. Finally, however, Morpheus was released and Sisyphus was sent to Tartarus, a particularly unpleasant region of Hades. There his punishment was that he had to push a boulder up to the top of the mountain and when he had just reached the summit the boulder would roll to the foot creating huge clouds of dust which obscured the light. Coughing and cursing, Sisyphus had to repeat the procedure through all eternity. Many writers, such as Camus (1942), have taken this to be the paradigm of a life of poor quality.

Let us now develop the myth to bring out some points relevant to our discussion of quality of life. Let us suppose that the demigod of medicine, Asklepios, pleads with Zeus to have some changes made in the punishment. First, he arranges that the boulder will no longer cause huge clouds of dust. As a result there are improvements to the lungs of Sisyphus and his health improves. Has his quality of life also been improved? Clearly it has. We therefore have one obvious factor in a good quality of life—health. Secondly, Asklepios arranges for some friends to visit Sisyphus to comfort him, wipe away the sweat, and so on. Has his quality of life been improved? Yes, loneliness diminishes quality of life and friends improve it. Thirdly, Asklepios persuades Zeus to transfer the place of punishment from the fearful environment of Tartarus to a Scottish mountain. He is still pushing the boulder, but in beautiful scenery. Once again, there is an improvement. Fourthly, the myth stresses the pointlessness of Sisyphus' activity. Let us suppose that Asklepios manages to modify the punishment further, so that Sisyphus now carries up different boulders and eventually succeeds in building a cairn, or even a shelter, at the top of the mountain. The activity now has a point, a minor creative purpose, and immediately we can say that there has been an improvement in quality of life. Fifthly, it is further agreed that Sisyphus will be allowed to abandon his boulder-pushing to help climbers whenever they may get into difficulties on the mountain. He now has an outlet for some skills and moral capacities, and we could perhaps claim that an outlet for moral qualities seems to improve quality of life. Sixthly, let us suppose that Sisyphus is allowed the occasional remission from his punishment—he is given every second weekend off or the like, during which period he can do other things. Once again we have an important factor in a good quality of life—some leisure and the possibility of varied activity. Finally, and most controversially, let us imagine an essential change. The original punishment was to go on through all eternity. Suppose that Asklepios pleads with Zeus about the everlasting nature of the sentence, and Zeus says, 'Okay I will allow him to die after one more year!' Does this improve his quality of life? Opinions might differ here. Some people might say that life is good whatever the quality. Indeed, if the life of Sisyphus has been improved under the six headings just mentioned, some people might say that it cannot possibly constitute a further improvement that this life will come to an end. Others might say that, whatever its quality, human life is by its very nature a transient affair. Indeed, it might be argued that a necessary condition of life's having meaning, or that what makes the very idea of quality possible, is that death comes to us all in the end; death supplies the framework or the parameters within which we can talk of meaning and quality. Let us assume the latter position for the moment because it enables us to bring to a close one particular type of analysis of 'quality of life'. We shall call it the 'significant toil' model of quality of life.

This model has the following features. It assumes that a life of good quality can be described under a number of headings: health, friends, environment, creativity, moral expression, leisure, an inevitable end. But three qualifications must be made of this picture. First, a life might be said to have a good quality, or a reasonable quality, even if not all seven elements are present. Secondly, there may be other similar headings which we have omitted; the headings are not necessarily exclusive. Thirdly, the headings must be interpreted in a flexible manner. For example, health is not an all-or-nothing matter, and some people stress their health more than others do. Again, for some people their creativity is in their employment and for others it is found in their leisure. Again, for some people friends are important while for others it might be a sexual partner or children. But with sympathetic interpretation of the headings we have a plausible model: a life of significant toil with death the signature of its completion. The life of good quality is here synonymous with the meaningful life, the valuable life, or the worthwhile life.

Why is this model plausible? The answer is that it taps into an important and widespread set of assumptions about human life, assumptions which go back to Greek mythology and are still present in all of us. They are that we all have something which can be called an essential human nature, and that it can be developed or realized or educated, granted the appropriate conditions. These assumptions, originally Greek, passed into Christian thought, where they were reinforced by the idea of God creating human beings in the divine image, that is with an essential nature.

Despite the plausibility of the significant toil model, however, it is open to four serious objections, each of which can give rise to a rival model of the quality of life, and thereby indirectly to a rival of the value of life. These are the choice model, the happiness model, the social needs model, and the culture model.

14.4 Choice

The origins of this objection can be found in the philosophy of Kant, and the Enlightenment more generally. It is that our description of the life of Sisyphus, even as improved by Asklepios, lacks one important ingredient, some would say the vital ingredient, for a life of good quality—choice. Sisyphus is compelled to push his boulder and the modifications of his punishment are all arranged on his behalf by Asklepios; he is totally without any choice. For Enlightenment thinkers this would be a fatal flaw in the significant toil model. In a political context it would be seen as 'enlightened despotism', and in a medical context it would be seen as 'beneficent paternalism'. Even such thinkers as the existentialists, who reject some enlightenment assumptions, would still insist on the central importance of choice. And the more extreme 'post-modernists', who reject all enlightenment assumptions, would still hold on to individual preference as expressed through choice as the most important or indeed the only factor making up a good quality of life. In health care ethics this point of view is strongly held and is expressed via the concept of autonomy. As we have seen in various previous contexts, the rhetoric of autonomy is all-pervasive in health care ethics, patients' movements, and the like.

How plausible is this objection and the alternative it offers? In general terms, for most people the framework of life, the boulder-pushing, is thrust upon them. If there is freedom or autonomy, it is within the framework which our situations in life, our heredity and environments, have determined. In terms of the myth, Sisyphus might decide which route to take up the mountain or what to do on his day off, and so it is for many people; we cannot really choose our lives. Within the more specific context of health care the reality can perhaps be expressed in two propositions: that it is the duty of the doctor, and the team, to provide an appropriate amount of information to the patient in a sensitive manner, and that patients are fully entitled to refuse their consent to any proposed treatment. Beyond that, the idea of patient autonomy is an illusion, and a dangerous one at that.

Nevertheless, let us develop further the idea of choice or autonomy as the central quality which makes life valuable. Supposing Zeus decides to release Sisyphus after many years of punishment and gives him a sum of money to help him back to ordinary life. Sisyphus proceeds to spend this money on whatever is the mythological equivalent of gambling machines, lottery tickets, scratch cards, and so on. Let us say he is successful, and makes an income from gambling. Has his quality of life been improved from the point at which he was pushing boulders to build shelters at the top of a pleasant mountain with his friends, and so on? If it is said that the single most important factor in quality of life is an individual's own preference expressed through choice, then it must follow that this life does have a better quality than the other, because to be a self is solely to be able to choose. This is the post-modern view of quality of life; agents are the only authorities on their own quality of life.

The particular health care exemplification of this view occurs when patients are seen as the only authorities on their treatments, regardless of effectiveness or cost. Patient autonomy is the single overriding value. This is a widespread view, which we reject (see Chapter 13, Section 13.2).

14.5   Happiness or well-being

A second criticism of the 'significant toil' model is that it does not mention the happiness of Sisyphus ('well-being' is the term more frequently used in health care writings but the problems are similar with both terms). According to this criticism, people's quality of life is solely their happiness or well-being.

One difficulty here is that 'happiness' and 'well-being' are ambiguous expressions. For the Greeks human nature has a certain structure, and happiness consists in developing content to the structure, or in acting in ways which express the form of that nature. Aristotle speaks of 'eudaimonia', a term which is translated as 'happiness' but really means 'living well and doing well'. It would follow from Aristotle's view of happiness that the life of significant toil is a happy life, even if it is not chosen. A second view of happiness sees it as success in obtaining the things that someone might want or choose. As the seventeenth century philosopher Thomas Hobbes (1651) puts it, the state of felicity is 'continual success in obtaining those things which a man, from time to time, desireth'. If this view of the nature of happiness is taken, then the second model of quality of life—the choice or autonomy model—can equally be described as a 'happiness' model.

But there is a third view of happiness—and it may be the dominant one in contemporary culture—which we can call the 'nice feelings' sense of happiness. The historical origins of this widespread view are in the writings of Jeremy Bentham (1789). According to this view we are happy if we are in certain states or moods in which pleasant feelings dominate. These moods have many variants or subsets, such as euphoria, bliss, exhilaration, rapture, or ecstasy, but common to all are powerful subjective feelings of pleasure. In the first model of happiness a person cannot be called happy unless activities are being undertaken which express or develop the self, and in the second a person cannot be happy unless they are choosing, but on the 'nice feelings' account a person can be called happy regardless of the causal origins of the feelings. For example, let us return to the myth of Sisyphus and imagine that Asklepios puts Sisyphus on a course of pills—Prozac or the like. We can imagine that Sisyphus is still undergoing his original punishment of pushing his boulder up the dusty mountain to be faced eternally with the futility of what he is doing. The myth describes him as groaning and cursing the gods. He is then put on the pills and as a result he becomes euphoric and brimming with nice feelings which totally divert him from the unending futility of his activities. Has his quality of life been improved? If happiness consists of nice feelings, regardless of their causation, and if quality of life consists of happiness in this sense, then the Prozac (or whatever) has indeed vastly improved quality of life. And it would follow that the quality of life of all of us might be improved if there were a drug which enhanced our feelings regardless of the grim reality of our actual situations.

In health care the situation described in the myth is far from uncommon. Imagine, for example, the many cases like that of the single mother living in damp housing in an area of multiple deprivation. The temptation for the GP to prescribe an antidepressant must be overwhelming. If we accept this as a valid account of 'quality of life' then quality of life can be improved although the life lived remains exactly as it was before. It is simply the patient's feelings which have changed. It is easy to see here how doctors can be described by unsympathetic socialists as 'agents of social control'. They are providing opiates for the masses which blind the poor to the reality of their social situations. Nevertheless, it is often said that your quality of life is just how you happen to be feeling. This view of quality is a rival to the first two models, for according to this view neither self-development nor choice is necessary for a good quality of life. Indeed, self-development and choice might interfere with the nice feelings in which this kind of quality of life consists.

14.6 Society and material needs

All three models of quality of life so far discussed could be criticized as being too individualistic. It might be said to be unrealistic—economically, politically, culturally, and even in terms of human nature—to base an account of quality of life simply round the individual. For example, take the opportunity costs. If a society puts a lot of money towards the problems of one person or one group of patients, then, by the same token, it has so much less to spend on other persons or groups. This has both a micro and a macro aspect. From the micro aspect we are thinking of a given health budget; if a large sum is spent on, say, chemotherapy then there is that much less to spend on the mentally handicapped. From the macro aspect we are thinking of the amounts which should be allocated to health as compared with education, housing, transport, and so on. Problems of this sort were discussed in our chapter on resource allocation. Again, the acid rain from the industry of one country will affect the quality of life of another country, so there is an international dimension to quality of life considerations. Moreover, there is a temporal dimension to this. Society is an entity which continually evolves through time, and the actions of one generation have a bearing on those of another. The material satisfactions of the future lay a claim on the political spenders of the present.

If we think of quality of life in this way two points are important. First, we are seeing quality of life in terms of the satisfaction of material needs, and secondly we are stressing human interrelatedness. The quality of life of one person has a bearing on that of another, and in health care in particular huge costs are potentially and actually involved. The ethical concept which should govern the supply of our health needs in this respect is equity. We are arguing that a full and adequate discussion of quality of life seen in a social perspective cannot be divorced from consideration of equity.

It is important to distinguish between equality and equity. The two words are often used interchangeably in relation to health and health care, yet they have different meanings. For example, women live longer than men due to biological differences. This is an inequality, but it is not inequitable. In other words, equality and inequality do not necessarily have an ethical basis, whereas equity always has an ethical basis because it concerns outcomes resulting from choice and opportunity. In discussing quality of life issues from a social perspective it is equity which is the relevant concept. Discussions of quality of life resulting from health care are sometimes distorted because they omit the social dimension to quality of life with its egalitarian claims. If quality of life is discussed from the point of view of the political left, then it must be seen in terms of society and cannot be adequately analysed on an individualistic basis.

14.7 Society and culture

But there is more to the quality of life of a society than health care, welfare, and social provision, no matter how equitably distributed. There is also what we might very broadly call the culture of a society—its architecture, science, public gardens, wildernesses, its consciousness of its history and heritage, its political cartoons, the accessibility of its art galleries and concert halls to the general public, and so on. What is necessary for the quality of life of a society is that its members should recognize that there are two different ways in which quality of life can be promoted. One is through health, welfare, and related goods, and here we should not be individualistic but thoroughly egalitarian. As long as we confine ourselves to this, however, we are acting as if health and material satisfaction are the only goods. But there is another side to quality of life which involves the promotion of ideals which are impersonal, yet are nevertheless essential to the dignity of a society and its flourishing through time. Indeed, they constitute our social identity. The quality of life of a society from this perspective assumes the position that some qualities are better than others, regardless of what is democratically chosen at a given point in history.

In sum, we have offered five different ways of looking at quality of life: as an individual life of significant toil, or of autonomous choice, or of subjective feelings of well-being, as a social life in which there is an equitable distribution of health and welfare, and as a social life in which the service of ideals of the good life are promoted alongside health and welfare.

14.8 Incommensurability and scales

The different ways of looking at quality of life can yield very different conclusions in different situations of health care, even more so in a broader social perspective. For example, the sufferer from Altzheimer's disease who is clean, fed, and watered may do well on the 'happiness' model of quality of life, but very badly on the 'significant toil' or choice model. Again, a political society with a high degree of health and welfare provision may do well on that way of looking at society, but may be criticized as a 'nanny state' because it does not stress individual choice and its accompanying responsibility, or cultural ideals. This makes it impossible to combine all the models into a single measure for evaluating health care. For a scale of any kind to be meaningful there must be an agreed unit of measurement. In other words, scientific measurement is inherently reductivist—concerned with one type of entity only— whereas quality of life is multifactorial, and the factors are inherently incommensurable, no matter how complex the mathematics. Hence, the attempt to produce 'quality of life scales' is bound to fail (Macnaughton 1996b).

The impossibility of producing meaningful scales in qualitative research has not deterred researchers from trying to create such scales. The attempts are inspired by the belief among medical researchers that nothing is truly scientific unless it involves measurement. Hence there has been a widespread attempt to quantify qualitative research. Let us take an example of such an attempt. Suppose a researcher is interested in the quality of the interaction between doctor and patient. If this quality is to be quantified then the researcher must pick some characteristics of the interview which are countable. Let us suppose that the researcher decides on, say, eye contact. No doubt eye contact can be counted (and perhaps someone has devised an eye contact scale!) but what would that show? Some patients might think it a good thing if their doctor keeps looking at them, but others may feel embarrassed or frightened. And the more discerning may become irritated at becoming the object of non-spontaneous behaviour, learned perhaps at a course on communication skills. The point is that doctor–patient or nurse–patient interviews ought to be holistic—one person responding to another in whichever way is comfortable to him or her—whereas whatever is quantifiable must be reductivist—in terms of specific characteristics, such as the angle of the chair, the respective levels of interviewer and interviewee, eye contact, and so on. But holistic human relationships cannot be reduced to a set of learned, measurable, behaviour patterns.

If this is true of professional–patient interviews, it is all the more true of much wider concepts such as quality of life. Quality of life is a holistic concept, so that whatever a researcher measures it would still be open to a patient to say 'What you have measured has nothing to do with my quality of life'.

The upshot of the discussion of quality of life is that as it is used in medicine it attempts to combine in one concept basically incompatible ingredients. Ideally, it should be discarded. What should be substituted are two different types of evaluation. First, the patient should be asked two questions: 'How are you feeling?' and 'Would you like the same treatment to continue?'. Secondly, the doctor should evaluate how far the medical goals are being achieved, how permanently, and at what cost. These two different types of evaluation can then be combined—and there is no mathematical way of doing this—and issued as the doctor's judgement, all things considered, including the patient's wishes.

14.9 The value of life

We can now return to the question of the value of a life. How do the models of quality of life affect our view on the value of life?

In terms of the first model the value of a life consists in its possession of those qualities which human beings have always valued—their health, friends, contributions to the lives of others, variety of interests, environment, and so on. As those qualities disappear the value of the life will diminish until it is negligible. This interpretation of the value of life is well represented in our society. Someone lacking those human characteristics is regarded as 'just a vegetable', that is as lacking the qualities which give value to a life. In terms of the second model the value of a life consists in a person's ability to exercise autonomous choice; where that does not exist there can be no value. Our attitudes here can be seen, for example, when an embryo is not accorded any rights. Or, in palliative care, when the doctor gives in to the demands of the autonomous relatives against the interests of the non-autonomous patient. The third model—quality of life consists in happiness in the sense of feelings of pleasure and the absence of pain—sees the value of the life of an individual in that single factor. It will follow from this that the elderly demented, provided they are well cared for, have lives with as much value as the scientific or artistic genius. Models four and five of quality of life switch the focus from the individual to society. The view is that we cannot form a view of the value of life of an individual without also looking at the society in terms of its equity of provision, and its culture; the value of the life of an individual is to some extent derivative from that of the individual's society.

Seen in this way health and welfare are in the end a set of relationships among citizens. As Dan Beauchamp (1987) puts it:

Collective goods are ultimately a set of relationships among the citizens of a community, relationships in which the community as a whole participates to obtain desired benefits. These collective goods include aggregate states of welfare or wellbeing, including declining rates of disease and premature deaths; efforts to limit the resources society devotes to personal health services; shared and common access to a good like medical care to foster the sense of community and membership in the group itself. And finally, there are those highly important collective goods, shared or common beliefs and values.

What follows from this about the provision of medical treatments? Two important conclusions follow. First, the point of medical treatments is presumably to assist in restoring some of the abilities, qualities, or activities which typically make life valuable. But it does not follow from this that these treatments make a greater claim on the public expenditure than a range of other claims; and in particular it does not follow that the claims of any one individual for life-saving therapies must necessarily be met. The reason for this has nothing to do with values in the sense of personal preferences; it has everything to do with the ethics of distributive justice. Secondly, it does not follow from the fact that a person's life has no value to them or anyone else that it is all right to harm them. The reason once again has to do with ethics and not values.

The important distinction between values and ethics is that values are rooted in personal preferences (although 'personal preferences' is perhaps too mild an expression for the tenacity with which we hold on to these particular preferences) whereas ethics are rooted in interpersonal rules. Without ethics society cannot survive; a system of ethics is the foundation of society and is the basis of law. Values change through time, but ethics do not change to the same extent, for the good reason that ethics offer one sort of protection necessary for our survival. This can be clearly seen in one area of ethics— human rights. Human rights are the contemporary descendants of natural rights which in turn derive from ideas of natural law going back to the Greeks. For example, Aristotle (4th century BC) writes in *Rhetoric* (1373b4):

It will now be well to make a complete classification of just and unjust actions. We may begin by observing that they have been defined relatively to two kinds of law ... By the two kinds of law I mean particular law and universal law. Particular law is that which each community lays down and applies to its own members; this is partly written and partly unwritten. Universal law is the law of nature. For there really is, as every one to some extent divines, a natural justice and injustice that is binding on all men, even on those who have no association or covenant with each other. It is this that Sophocles' Antigone clearly means when she says that the burial of Polyneices was a just act in spite of the prohibition: she means that it was just by nature.

This passage, and there are many similar from the Greeks to the Declaration of Human Rights, witnesses to a deep-rooted sense in human beings of the overriding importance of some rules of morality or ethics, namely the basic ones necessary for a decent human life.

The point is sufficiently important to be worth expanding. It is natural for people to ask 'What is morality?' But if we remember Wittgenstein's account of the fly in the bottle (p. 289) we might find it more profitable to change the question and ask 'What is morality for?' In answering this question we can draw attention to certain features of human beings and our lives together in society, in any society. First, human beings are in various ways vulnerable to each other and to the environment. For example, we have bodies which require constant nourishment, warmth, and protection from disease and attack. In short, we have basic physical and psychological needs. That is why any culture has rules enjoining us not to harm each other and to help where possible. In a similar way, we are vulnerable psychologically. Consider, for example, the many ways in which people can hurt each other by slander, ingratitude, obscenity, patronizing behaviour, and so on. If any society is to survive, therefore, it requires rules of harmony, to smooth out as far as possible sources of conflict. Moreover, human needs and wants can be satisfied more easily by cooperative policies, such as are involved in the division of labour. This is especially important if we bear in mind that commodities are scarce and require labour to produce them. These features of the human situation—vulnerability, the need for harmony and cooperation, and the scarcity of commodities—are at the root of the whole area of social justice. If we add to this the facts that human knowledge and rationality are limited, and that mutual sympathy, while it exists in all of us, is also limited in its scope, we begin to see what morality, or ethics in the sense of morality, is for. It is to make life go a little better than it otherwise would, or it is to protect our lives, liberties, and happiness against threats from each other, the environment, and disease.

It can be seen from these features of human life, and the function which ethics has in making it go better than it otherwise would, why ethics does not change so much as 'values'. Values are in the end personal preferences, but ethics is a system of interpersonal rules for the better ordering of human life. That is why medicine ought not to abandon its traditional concern with ethics and chase after fashionable values such as 'advocacy' or 'holistic care'. Next year, the fashions may change. It may be this point which people have in mind when they say that life has an 'infinite value', but the point is better put in terms of ethics: it is that no one has a right to do away with a life, or negligently to harm it, even if it is lacking in value.

At the end of the day, then, the question of whether a given autonomous or a given non-autonomous human being does or does not have a life with a certain kind of quality or value has no direct bearing on the question of ethics or morality: whether that human being may or may not be killed by a physician or by anyone else, with or without consent. The latter question is indeed important, but it is not discussed directly by us because it is so widely discussed elsewhere, to the extent that members of the general public have gained one of two mistaken impressions: either that the sole purpose of the palliative care movement is to stop voluntary euthanasia ever becoming legal, or that the purpose of palliative care is covertly to carry out euthanasia!

Perhaps it is appropriate that we should conclude our book where we began, with the wise view of Dr Samuel Johnson (1755):

> *If the changes we fear be thus irresistible, what remains but to acquiesce with silence, as in the other insurmountable distresses of humanity? It remains that we retard what we cannot repel, that we palliate what we cannot cure.*

References

Adair, J. (1987). *Effective teambuilding*. Gower Publishing Co. Ltd.

Aristotle (4th century BC). *Nicomachean ethics* (trans. W. D. Ross 1925). Oxford University Press.

Aristotle (4th century BC). *Rhetoric* (ed. R. Mckeon 1941). Random House, New York.

British Medical Association (1995). *Advance statements about medical treatment: code of practice with explanatory notes*. Report of the British Medical Association. BMJ Publishing Group, London.

Beauchamp, D. (1987). Life-style, public health and paternalism. In *Ethical dilemmas in health promotion* pp. 69–82 (ed. S. Doxiadis). Wiley, Chichester.

Beauchamp, T. L. and Childress, J. F. (1994). *Principles of biomedical ethics*, 4th edn. Oxford University Press.

Bentham, J. (1789). *Principles of morals and legislation*. Oxford University Press.

Brewin, T. (1998). Wasted words. *Journal of the Royal College of Physicians of London*, **32**, (4), 333–4.

Camus, A. (1942). *The myth of Sisyphus*. Gallimard, Paris.

Department of Health (1991). Local research ethics committees. In *Health service guidelines*. NHS Management Executive (HSG (91) 5), Department of Health, London.

Department of Health (1995). *The Patient's Charter and you*. HMSO, London.

Downie, R. S. and Calman, K. C. (1994). *Healthy respect: ethics in health care*. Oxford University Press.

Downie, R. S. and Charlton, B. (1992). *The making of a doctor*. Oxford University Press.

Doyle, D., Hanks, G. W. C., and MacDonald, N. (eds) (1994). *Oxford textbook of palliative medicine*. Oxford University Press, New York.

Hobbes, T. (1651). *Leviathan* (ed. C. B. Macpherson 1968). Penguin Books, Harmondsworth.

Hurwitz (1998). *Clinical guidelines and the law: negligence, discretion and judgment*. Radcliffe Medical Press, Abingdon.

Hutcheson, F. (1725). *An inquiry into the origin of our ideas of beauty and virtue* (ed. R. S. Downie 1994). Everyman Library, London.

Jonsen, A. R. (1990). *The new medicine and the old ethics*. Harvard University Press, Cambridge, MA.

Kant, I. (1785). *Fundamental principles of the metaphysics of ethics* (ed. H. J. Paton 1948). Hutchinson, London.

Law Commission (1995). *Report on mental incapacity* 6.29, 6.34, 6.36. Law Commission, London.

Lewis, C. S. (1942). *The screwtape letters*. Pan Books, London.

Macnaughton, J. (1996a) Anecdote in clinical practice. In *Narrative based medicine* (ed. T. Greenhalgh and B. Hurwitz). BMJ Books, London.

Macnaughton, J. (1996b). Numbers, scales and qualitative research. *Lancet*, **347**, 1099–100.

McQuay, H. and Moore, A. (1994). Need for rigorous assessment of palliative care. *British Medical Journal*, **309**, 1315–6.

McWhinney, I. R., Bass, M. J., and Donner, A. (1994). Evaluation of a palliative care service: problems and pitfalls. *British Medical Journal*, **309**, 1340–2.

Mill, J. S. (1859). *On liberty* (ed. M. Warnock 1962). Collins, London.

Paris, J. J., Schreiber, M. D., Statter, M., Arensman, R., and Seigler, M. (1993). Sounding board. *New England Journal of Medicine*, **329**, (5), 354–7.

Pellegrino, E. D. and Thomasma, D. C. (1988). *For the patient's good: the restoration of beneficence in health care*. Oxford University Press.

Pellegrino, E. D. and Thomasma, D. C. (1993). *The virtues in medical practice*. Oxford University Press, New York.

Percival, T. (1803). *Medical ethics* (ed. C. Leake 1976), p. 71. Krieger, New York.

R v Adams (1957). *Criminal Law Review*, p. 365.

Re J. (a minor) (1992). 4 *All England Reports*, 614. For discussion, see 'British judges cannot order doctors to treat'. *Hastings Centre Report* 1992, **22**, (4), 3–4.

Rogers, C. (1969). *On becoming a person: a therapist's view of psychotherapy*. Constable, London.

Royal College of Physicians (1990). *Guidelines on the practice of ethics committees in medical research involving human subjects*. Royal College of Physicians, London.

Veatch, R. M. and Spicer, C. M. (1992). Medically futile care; the role of the physician in setting limits. *American Journal of Law and Medicine*, **18**, 15–36.

Wesley, S. (1996). The rise of counselling and the return of alienism. *British Medical Journal*, **313**, 158–60.

Wilkes, E. (1989). In *Doctors' decisions: ethical conflicts in medical practice* (ed. G. R. Dunstan and E. A. Shinebourne), Ch. 19, p. 199. Oxford University Press, New York.

Wittgenstein, L. (1953). *Philosophical investigations*. Blackwell, Oxford.

Index